SHOULDER PAIN

FIX THE SYSTEM TO FIX THE SYMPTOMS

HOW TO USE TOTAL MOTION RELEASE (TMR) TO GET RID OF YOUR SHOULDER PAIN FOR GOOD

CHIP MOSELEY, MPT

COPYRIGHT © 2022 CHIP MOSELEY

ALL RIGHTS RESERVED

CONTENTS

Introduction		3
Chapter 1	How Shoulder Pain Can Dramatically Affect Your Life	7
Chapter 2	The Three Most Common Reactions to Shoulder Pain That Often Do Not Work	11
Chapter 3	Is There Hope For Me? How Can I Know?	17
Chapter 4	What Is the Rotator Cuff?	23
Chapter 5	What Causes Shoulder Pain?	27
Chapter 6	How Tightness of the Body Causes Shoulder Pain	35
Chapter 7	Share the Workload and Work the Power Zones	43
Chapter 8	Do I Need an X-ray or MRI Before I Consider Starting Any Treatment Program?	51
Chapter 9	The Five Most Common Shoulder Injuries	55
Chapter 10	Common Treatment Options Outside of Therapy	65
Chapter 11	Why Traditional Exercise Can Make You Worse	69
Chapter 12	How to Know If Treatment Is Working – The Secret of the "TREAT"	75
Chapter 13	Introduction to TMR (Total Motion Release) – A Better Option	83
Chapter 14	Chip's Four Favorite Exercises for Shoulder Pain Patients	105
Chapter 15	How Long Does It Take To Get My Shoulder Better? Will the Exercise Benefits Last?	131
Chapter 16	What Treatment Looks Like in Our Clinic	145
Chapter 17	Summarizing It All – A Review of the Key Principles	149
Chapter 18	Success Stories	153
About the Author		157

INTRODUCTION

Do you struggle with shoulder pain? The kind that seems to linger on and never get better? The kind that makes it hard to sleep at night and lift your arm over your head? If yes, know that I am writing this book for you. Why am I doing this? The answer to that question is very simple.

This book about shoulder pain is about empowerment. This empowerment comes from knowledge I will bestow, as well as effective actionable treatments that you can do to yourself. I want to give you the tools on how to understand your shoulder problem and how to fix it for good. These fixes will also be natural and organic through your own body movements and not using medications, injections, or surgery.

This book is for those of you that are stuck in the pain cycle of going through long periods of suffering. You have pain. Then you seek out treatment or rest the arm for a period of time. You think you are starting to improve. Then later on, the problem just comes back again. And again. And again. Or possibly maybe you are the one that has never had any moments of relief at all.

You can tell that as time goes on longer with this pain, the problem has become more and more difficult to handle. The treatments that helped even slightly before do not seem to help as much now. What was short-term relief doing a certain treatment is no longer offering you even short-term gains. And you want long-term gains. You are tired of seeing many doctors, therapists, pharmacists, and others for this issue. You want it fixed and fixed now!

So you may ask, "How is this book going to be any different for me?" Especially if you feel like you have heard it all and met every type of clinician that treats shoulder issues without ever having any sustainable success.

First of all, up front, I am a physical therapist by profession and training. I am also the owner of a physical therapy company in Raleigh, NC named Total Motion Physical Therapy. We have seen countless shoulder patients since we opened in the late 1990s. Other than back pain, shoulder pain issues are the second most common problem we have seen over the last few decades. However, if you just look over the last two years in our clinic, shoulder pain has actually become the #1 most common pain problem we treat in the clinic.

Just in case you are wondering if this is your "typical" physical therapist perspective on shoulder pains....think again! Maybe you have been to physical therapy before, just to find that those traditional treatments did not work at all for you. If anything, you felt only short-term gains or even worse for having attended those painful appointments.

In the following chapters, I will describe for you what first causes these shoulder problems. I bet you will be surprised to find out the real reason why people get shoulder pains is not what you may have heard before. I will go over the typical responses and treatment options that do not work to fix the problem for the longer term. We will explore the anatomy and different types of shoulder diagnoses. Then after all of that information, I will show you a way to view the body and treat your shoulder pain in a manner that you probably have never tried before. And I will give you 4 specific treatments to try using those new techniques.

Our clinic, Total Motion PT, is also the alpha site for an amazing tool on how to fix pains called TMR, short for Total Motion Release. This tool was created at our clinic two decades ago specifically to empower patients to fix their own pains. We often like to say, "Treat yourself to pain relief"! I will introduce you to the beginnings of a brand new skill for you to fix your shoulder pain for good using only what God gave you. No medications, surgeries, or fancy machines needed. Not even a hot or cold pack. All you need is your own body and some important knowledge on how to use it for healing. This is great news! You can do all of these natural fixes for yourself. All you have to do is move your body in planned, specific ways to fix your pain.

I look forward to going on this journey with you through this book.

Special thanks and gratitude are owed to:

1. The Lord Jesus Christ, who creates our bodies with the mechanisms on how to maximize the healing process when we learn how to listen to the feedback it gives.
2. My amazing and beautiful wife of three decades, Nancy, who supports me in all I do. You will always be the favorite person in my life.

3. Tom Dalonzo-Baker, the founder of this tool TMR, which we will discuss in this book. I am thankful how Tom got me and our clinic started on this amazing journey. We have created a tool on how to fix not only pains, but also how to fix the cause of these pains for good in a manner never created before.

CHAPTER ONE

HOW SHOULDER PAIN CAN DRAMATICALLY AFFECT YOUR LIFE

A few months back, I met this nice lady, whom I will call Jill for the sake of this book. She came to our physical therapy clinic here in Raleigh for help with her severe shoulder pain. The first words out of her mouth were not even any form of "Hello." Instead, she walked straight up to me and said, "My right shoulder and arm pain is so severe that I can't even sleep at night! When I roll to either side, especially on the right side, the pain is so high I can't even stand it! Have you ever heard of this before?"

I answered her that pain with laying down is extremely common with shoulder injuries. Actually, it is probably the number one complaint from those who are suffering with these problems. It is understandably frustrating to have limited sleep due to that problem. Life is much less happy when we are not well rested. Healing is also much slower without proper rest. She also continued to list pain and limitations with several other actions below.

- Reaching overhead
- Reaching to the back seat of her car
- Lifting heavier items like a jug of milk
- Exercising at the gym
- Getting her shirt on and off
- Putting on deodorant

- Doing her hair
- Scratching her back
- Putting on her bra
- Making a meal

She leaned over and whispered to me so no one else in the clinic could hear and said, "My pain can be so bad that I can't even wipe myself when I go to the bathroom. You have to help me!"

The good news is that Jill noticed that she could begin to feel better even on her first session. Then just about five weeks later, after our treatment plan, she reported feeling 100% pain free with everything she wanted to do. She got her life back again and is back to feeling like her normal self again.

Now let's take this back to you...

Can you relate with Jill?

Maybe you do not have every single problem on her list of limitations, but do you struggle with at least with some of those actions she struggled with? Like laying on that arm or reaching overhead? Maybe you have your own list of difficulties and goals, in addition to what she mentioned as her symptoms.

Maybe you cannot hold your baby or grandbaby without fear of pain or even dropping the child. Or possibly you cannot play ball, tennis, or do that fun activity with friends that you used to love doing all the time. Or throw a ball to your child.

Even the basic tasks of life that we take for granted can be severely affected by a shoulder injury. For some of you, this pain and limitation can go on for months, years, and even decades without relief.

Over the last few years, I have also realized how the mind-body-spirit connection is in effect as well. If you physically feel poor, it also affects how you feel about other areas of life. Maybe your physical pain trickles in to how you treat your spouse, kids, coworkers, parents, friends, or others. You can get frustrated with pain and then treat them poorly so now those relationships are strained. This emotional strain and stress then also lead us to be more physically strained even further. Then that cycle can feed itself for years, making it harder and harder to get out of the hole that has been created. Physical problems affect the mind and spirit negatively. Which in turn makes the physical problem worse. It goes on and on.

How do you get out of that cycle?

We are going to address this throughout the book.

Key Thought #1: Shoulder pain can severely affect how you enjoy life. Seeking out proper treatment quickly is critical to getting your life back.

CHAPTER TWO

THE THREE MOST COMMON REACTIONS TO SHOULDER PAIN THAT OFTEN DO NOT WORK

Can you relate to Jill from the previous chapter? You know that you need to get better. You want to get your life back to normal again. The problems have become so severe that your body is screaming at you to do something about it.

However, you may be wondering what the smartest course of action of treatment is for your problem. Let me ask you this question. What do you think the majority of people choose to do when this problem first starts to occur, even if the pain is severe? What do you tend to do first when you have muscle and joint pains?

The most common first reaction is typically **just to do nothing** with the hope that the problem goes away with time. To be fair, I can relate to this decision to just ignore the problem. I am a father of five children. Over the years, I have been "coach" for many teams. I have been a Sunday School teacher for a few decades. I own a physical therapy company which includes treating patients 40 hours a week as well as other owner related tasks. I have been married to the most beautiful and wonderful wife in the world for twenty-eight years who also needs my attention as well. All these things take up a lot of time in the week.

I do not have time to be hurt. If I was injured, where would I find the time to take care of myself?

So what do we tend to do? We wait until the problem crosses that line of severity to where it makes us HAVE TO DEAL WITH IT. Unfortunately, by that time, the problem has progressed to a place where it is much, much harder to fix than if you had addressed it earlier on. This is true in many areas of life. Problems with family, work or friends can be ignored until they reach a boiling point. Then fixing those issues can take months or years. It would have been so much easier to just fix it in the earlier stages. Ignoring is bad.

A couple of years ago, my wife informed me on a Tuesday morning that I had a physical scheduled for 10:00 a.m. at our doctor's office. I told her I had not scheduled any such appointment. She told me that she knew that I would not make such an appointment myself, so she scheduled it for me because she loves me. In her defense, my previous physical prior to that was back in the 1990s. I just turned fifty this year. So yes, I was due. However, the good news is that I checked out pretty well and I went home and told my wife that "I guess I can wait another twenty years until my next physical, right"! To which she looked at me with her beautiful, hazel eyes and then proceeded to roll them back into her head.

Can you relate with me, though? Ignoring the pain and hoping it gets better with time is a very common mistake. This is the number one problem we see when it comes to shoulder problems. By not addressing the issue quickly, the injury goes deeper and often becomes more severe, potentially even leading to soft tissue tears or other more severe forms of damage. The deeper the problem, the longer it takes to fix. If ignoring the problem and hoping time fixes it is the number one mistake, what is number two?

The second most common mistake starts when you feel the problem is severe enough that you actually decide to seek out help from your doctor. Most of the time when a patient goes to his/her primary doctor and discusses shoulder pain, what do you think the average doctor chooses for your treatment? Consult with an orthopedic surgeon? Physical therapy? Give you a sheet of exercises to perform? Possibly. But those choices by far are not the most common action taken by primary care doctors on such initial appointments. So what do they do? Typically, that patient is sent home with a **prescription anti-inflammatory or steroid medication**, right?

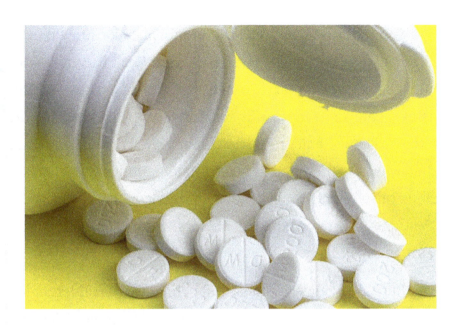

So the second most common mistake that is made for those in shoulder pain is to drug the problem. We will discuss the mechanics of what causes shoulder problems to occur in the first place later in this book. Medications do not ever change the mechanics of what causes a shoulder problem. They can help the pain and inflammation go down to some degree, for a certain period of time. This does have value. However, if you do not fix the mechanical cause, the problem will continue to get worse and worse over time.

What is the third most common mistake after ignoring the problem and trying to drug the problem away? I will give you a hint. In addition to the medication you received from your primary care doctor, what is the next recommendation you get from that doc? The next action typically is to send the shoulder pain patient to an **orthopedic surgeon for a consult**.

Some may be surprised that this is a mistake. I might even have some great doctors in town reading my book right now who would be surprised that I would include this action in the "mistake" category. Orthopedic surgeons serve a great purpose in health care and shoulder injuries. I am very thankful they exist and do what they do. There are also shoulder injuries that are of such severity, that I myself would immediately refer these patients to those orthopedic doctors before beginning any treatment in our clinic.

But ask yourself, statistically do most shoulder pains require surgery at first? The answer of course is no. What do orthopedic surgeons do? They mostly do surgery and injections. Injections are just a deeper form of oral medications. Again, the injections are not fixing the problem and the surgery is not needed as of yet. So who would those surgeons send that patient to in order to try to address the mechanics and pain of the nonsurgical shoulder pain problem? We will discuss this later on in the book. It would have been more efficient to bypass the primary care doctor and orthopedic surgeon and just directly go to the person that is the most appropriate to address the most common problems. This saves time and money in the process. The earlier you get the proper help, the easier the pain is to fix.

Quick review. The three most common mistakes people make with shoulder pain early on are to:

- Wait and do nothing, ignoring the issue and hoping time fixes it

- Try to drug the problem with oral medications and injections
- Seek out the care of an orthopedic surgeon when surgery is not needed yet

So if you do not presently need or want surgery and you do not want to keep ignoring and drugging your shoulder problem, what other options do you have? The best option is to fix not only the symptoms but also the root cause of the problem. We will discuss later what I mean by this root cause. Fixing is good. But you need to have the right tools.

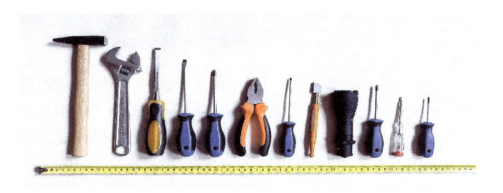

Key Thought #2: Choosing the wrong treatment or waiting longer to address the problem can make the shoulder injury worse and more difficult to properly treat.

CHAPTER THREE

IS THERE HOPE FOR ME? HOW CAN I KNOW?

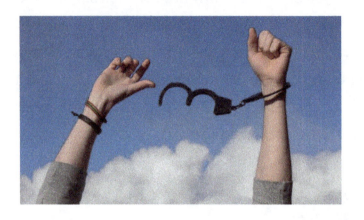

Let's say that you are not the person who made the mistakes of the last chapter. You didn't just ignore the problem. You didn't want to just try to fix the pain with medications and injections. You didn't feel the need to see a surgeon when one was not needed yet.

Maybe you have already tried a variety of actions that at first made sense and sounded positive.

You got an X-ray.

You got an MRI.

You tried physical therapy.

You tried massage.

You went to the gym and tried to strengthen your muscles.

You went to yoga and stretch classes.

You went to your chiropractor.

You even tried alternative treatments like acupuncture.

And yet, here you are!

You feel like you've tried EVERYTHING out there.

So should you give up hope? How could you know if there is still a chance that you could get back to normal?

One big factor that can tell you if there is hope, is when you realize that you have some degree of power and control over your pain. What do I mean by that control? For example, do you recognize that there are certain tasks in your day that seem to make the problem **WORSE**? Perhaps the pain gets worse with laying on the arm, lifting the arm, lifting items with weight, getting dressed, or other actions. You understand that your actions can make this pain go up and get worse. We do not like, of course, this pain to go up.

However, when you realize that you have the power to make the pain worse, then by contrast, logic that tells you that there are also actions you can do that make the **PAIN GO DOWN** as well. One way you can make the pain less is just to avoid the actions that make the pain worse. The other is to find those positive actions that promote healing.

If you have not yet had success finding those positive actions, it does not necessarily mean that such solutions do not exist. But you must stay away from ignoring "Einstein's definition of insanity", which to paraphrase means that you do not want to keep doing the same actions for treatment that you have done before that have proven not to fix your shoulder pains. You know that a certain prescription of actions did not work before. You need to find a different recipe and solution. If you have been to treatment of one kind for weeks and never found improvement of any kind, if you continued doing that same option for several more weeks, will it work then when it did not before? Probably not. Most chronic pain patients in treatment will usually have up and down moments and up and down days. But in your past or present courses of treatment, did you notice your healing trending on an average upward slope or were you staying the same or getting worse over time?

If you have a muscle or joint pain, there will be motions and physical activities that make the pain go up and down. You might lift a heavy weight and the pain gets worse. You might put the arm in a sling and it feels better. Contrast that with someone who says that their pain is EXACTLY THE SAME, ALL DAY, NO MATTER WHAT they seem to do. First of all, most of the time a patient makes this statement, it is not true. They just emotionally feel that life is hard right then and nothing seems to make it better. However, there are an extremely small percentage of patients who might have a pain that is not from muscles and joints. Examples would be like diseases of the lungs or other organs that could still present as muscle pain near the shoulder. So if you literally feel that you could raise your arm overhead a lot, lift weight, lay on that arm, and do other activities with your shoulder and your pain DOES NOT CHANGE OR GET WORSE but still have a high intensity long lasting shoulder pain, then you might want to visit your doctor and see if there are other medical issues to examine. But if your pain can get worse with certain motions and activities, and go down with certain motions or other activities, you have a musculoskeletal problem and there is hope for you.

Do not allow yourself to get stuck in a mindset that says that nothing can help you. If you have sought out help before and not had success, it is understandable that you could feel this way. However, this mindset is dangerous. Some people even look to blame their pains on excuses like bad genetics, the weather, a certain history, or other factors that they have no power to change. By blaming their problem on those factors, basically they are saying that they should not even try to get better since there is nothing that can help them to be any better. These excuses make you want to just accept your pain and not even try to do anything about it.

The Serenity Prayer Patient

I often talk about the "serenity prayer" patient. The paraphrased shorter version goes something like, "Lord, help me to change the things I have the power to change, accept the things I do not have the power to change, and have the wisdom to know which is which". It may be true that the problems can be worse from genetics, weather changes, or past events. **Lord, help me**

to accept those things. However, you might have the ability to change other factors like muscle tightness and weakness, the contribution into that painful area from other muscles and joints, diet, and other factors in your control. ***Lord, help me to change what I can change to help me with my shoulder pain.***

If your pain can go up, your pain can go down. Do not stop searching for your answer if you have not yet found it. The answer may just lie in something you have not tried yet. When I show you my favorite four exercises later in this book, I can almost guarantee that you have never tried those exercises before in the way I will show you. Hopefully at least one will change how you feel about your shoulder problem and give you hope.

Key Thought #3: If you can do actions that make the pain go up, then you have a musculoskeletal issue and there are actions you can do to make the pain go down.

CHAPTER FOUR

WHAT IS THE ROTATOR CUFF?

Our bodies are beautifully and wonderfully created. Shoulders, in particular, are extremely powerful joints that when healthy, have a large capacity for force and motion. However, we know from physics class, when you **INCREASE MOBILITY**, you **DECREASE STABILITY**. Since your shoulder joint has the capacity for great mobility, this increases the challenge on the joint to remain stable and keep the humerus in the socket. This means that the arm could easily come out of alignment, out of socket, and get injured unless some mechanism is put in place to keep all of the pieces held together. The rotator cuff is designed to give us motion while trying to hold the arm bone centered in the socket.

The rotator cuff is a group of four muscles and tendons that help to hold your arm bone, the **humerus**, in the center of the socket of your shoulder blade bone, called the **scapula**. These tissues also help in the creation of motion in your arm in all directions. They help not only to increase motion and speed with activities with the arm, but they also help to control the speed of your arm when it moves in order to keep that humerus properly connected to the socket without injury.

The four muscles and tendons that are part of the rotator cuff are named:

- Supraspinatus
- Infraspinatus
- Teres Minor
- Subscapularis

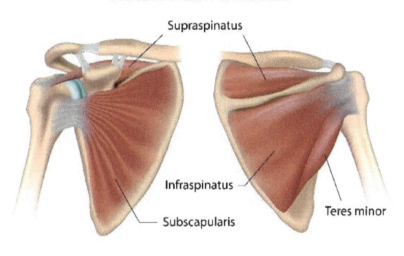

There are some who also want to include other ligaments and connective tissues in with their definitions of "rotator cuff". The shoulder has many ligaments, which are tissues that connect from one bone to another, that also are holding the bones together. The labrum is a thick piece of tissue that acts as an attachment site for certain ligaments and also makes the size of the cup of the shoulder joint functionally larger to add more stability. The ligaments and labrum are different from the muscles and tendons in that they do not have the ability to contract. All of these tissues can be injured and lead to pain and difficulty.

The three main bones we will discuss with the shoulder joint and use of the rotator cuff are:

- Humerus (arm bone)
- Scapula (shoulder blade)
- Clavicle (collar bone)

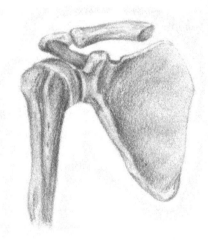

Key Thought #4: Understanding how the anatomy of the rotator cuff works will start you on the journey of knowing how to fix your shoulder pain.

CHAPTER FIVE

WHAT CAUSES SHOULDER PAIN?

Some injuries to the shoulder/rotator cuff can be due to trauma, like a fall or car accident. In our clinic, we find that these traumas are rarely ever the cause of the shoulder pains we treat. In fact, trauma make for less than 5% of our shoulder pain patients.

How about postures? Can they cause the shoulder pains? Poor posture can be an irritant to the shoulder joint. The more we slouch, the more we compress certain tendons and other tissues in between the bottom of tip of the outer edge of the shoulder blade and the top of my humerus. (See picture below).

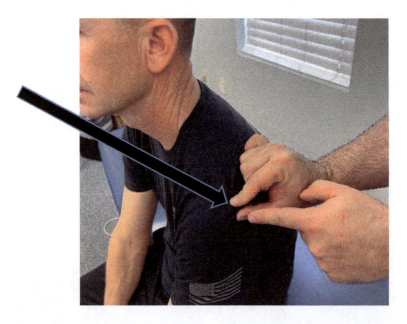

Furthermore, if we lay on that arm at night, the humerus bone is pushed up into that same space, which again adds pain through compressing certain tendons and ligaments.

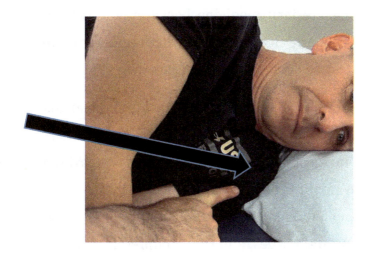

While postures can irritate these tissues, I still find that they are not typically the true cause of shoulder pain. If this was the case, then pretty much 100% of people who work on computers and slouch a bit and 100% of people who lay on their sides at night would have a high degree of shoulder pain. We do not see that is the case. But if you have someone who already is hurting or predisposed to shoulder dysfunctions, doing those postures of slouching and laying on the side adds to the pain and injury and makes proper healing even harder to occur.

The Surprising Real Cause of Shoulder Pain

If most shoulder pains are not caused by direct shoulder trauma or postures, where do the high majority of shoulder problems begin? Not sure of the answer? Well, let me help you to feel better. I know many doctors, physical therapists, and others who have no idea what the answer is to this question either. This is because the answer lies in places where we are often not trained to look. Even most medical schools and physical therapy schools, with our typical western medicine backgrounds, will not even teach how to properly find and treat what I am getting ready to teach you. So where does the shoulder pain begin?

Most shoulder injuries are due to wear and tear that force bones in the shoulder to compress together due to **TIGHTNESS,** throwing off the mechanics of how that shoulder was designed to move. So you might read this and think, that's not really that extraordinary of a thought, the shoulder gets tight and it squishes certain tendons and tissues, and that compression leads to pain, inflammation, and damage. Well, here's what you probably did not expect me to say. The real culprits are really the tightness of the muscles and joints **OUTSIDE OF THE SHOULDER ITSELF,** in other areas of the body.

Many of us are trained to imagine that we have this arm bone that is moving around in space by rotating on a still socket in our shoulder blade. To illustrate this in the picture below, imagine my measuring stick to be an arm bone and observe how that would pinch into the shoulder blade if it did not move out of the way.

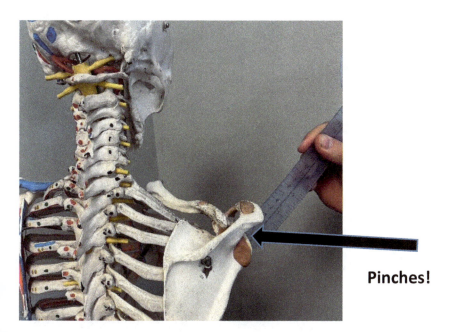

Pinches!

This is actually NOT what happens when we move with a healthy shoulder. In order to have proper functional use in our arms, when the humerus moves, the shoulder blade (scapula) and collar bone (clavicle) should also be moving along with the arm. So now observe the difference if the shoulder blade and collar bone are moving with the lifting of the "arm" represented by my measuring stick.

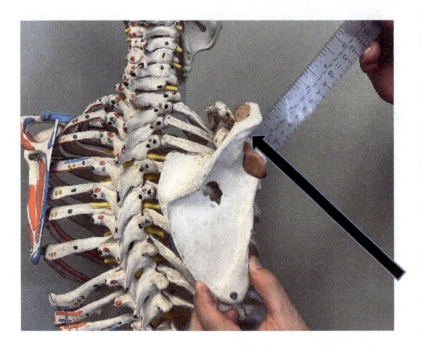

Less pinch when shoulder blade moves

If there is any **TIGHTNESS** anywhere in the body that keeps this scapula from moving at the same speed and flexibility as the arm bone is moving, then the edge of the scapula, called the acromion, does not "get out of the way" properly in time when the arm moves. This leads to **PINCHING** of those shoulder tissues and altering of how the humerus moves in the socket. In between the top of the humerus and the bottom of the acromion, in the space as shown in the picture below, we have a few tendons, ligaments, and bursae that do not like to be compressed and pinched in that manner.

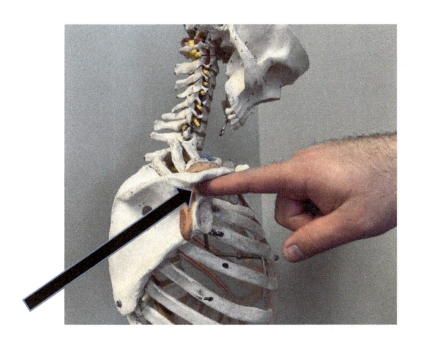

It is tightness that keeps the scapula and clavicle from moving properly that causes the shoulder to pinch and create these injuries. **So where does this tightness originate? What causes a tissue to get tight in the first place? Genetics, or something else?**

When the body has an injury moment, even if it is just brief one like falling on your butt in snow on your driveway, the body will tighten up those tissues around that area to protect it from further injury. It is very possible that in a short period of time, the pain actually does go away. But often the tightness is what remains in the system for a longer period of time. It is the tightness from these other joints and muscles elsewhere in the body that then changes how the arm moves. We will continue to build on this thought in the next chapter.

Key Thought #5: Shoulder pain is caused by tightness in the body that changes the mechanics of how the arm would normally move. This tightness can originate from any place in the body.

CHAPTER SIX

HOW TIGHTNESS OF THE BODY CAUSES SHOULDER PAIN

How does tightness in the other parts of the body lead to shoulder pain? To help illustrate this, I am going to give you a potentially horrific visual. I want you to imagine for a moment someone wearing a giant, super tight leotard. This leotard will go over the head like a tight Spiderman mask, extend into the chest, down the arms, down into the rest of the torso and all the way down through the legs and under the feet.

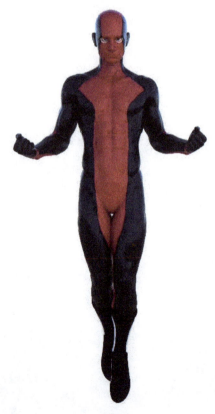

For your own benefit, there will be no attached picture in this book of me specifically wearing such an item. If you need a specific visual of a person, feel free to imagine this same leotard on yourself or on someone who is much better looking in your life. So what is this "leotard?" In anatomy class, we have several names for it. The leotard is made up of skin, connective tissue called fascia, ligaments, tendons, bone, muscles, fat, organs, and plenty of other tissues. The point is, **ALL THE PARTS OF THE BODY ARE CONNECTED.** Changes made to one part of the body cause changes to the tissues they connect with. This then creates a chain reaction of events even further into our bodies.

To help to illustrate how this leotard works, let's do this little simple exercise. While wearing a shirt, take one arm and reach it as high over your head as you can. If you have an injury, feel free to do this with your better arm that does not hurt as much for now. Reach high enough that not only your arm is raising, but you feel your ribs elevate, and your spine and hip feel stretched. Tune in to how high and how easy that felt to perform. See picture below for an example.

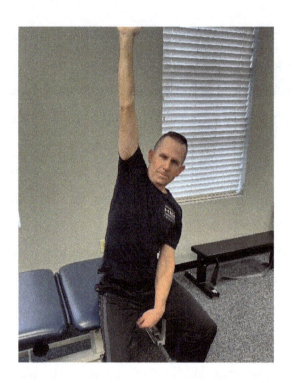

Keeping your hand on that shirt, now try to raise that same arm again. You will notice that you will be unable to raise the arm as high or as well as before.

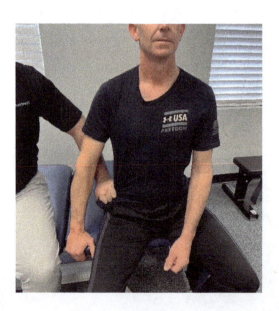

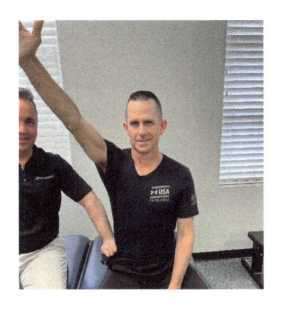

Originally this restriction might not cause shoulder pain but rather what looks more like tightness or a lack in range of motion. But given time with that restriction on this hip tightness example, this will actually lead to more pinching of those shoulder tendons and create shoulder injuries. So, in this case, what was the **CAUSE** of the shoulder injury? What caused this shoulder pinching? It was not the shoulder itself, but rather the hip tightness from below that made the shoulder pinch.

I have treated many patients over the years who have had multiple shoulder surgeries, seen multiple therapists and other clinicians, had countless medications and injections, and other treatments because "the shoulder pain" would not get better. Then after attending the first session, I explained to them how this tightness of the hip below their shoulder is the reason why they were never improving. The hip was holding the arm in its injury state. Then I give them a simple leg exercise that improved how well that hip moved. Then lo and behold, all of a sudden, it felt like magic; that shoulder pain of many years was dramatically lessened and improved in its motion and function! Often when this happens, the patient may say we just did some crazy voodoo trick on them. But that positive change really was just anatomy class joined with a physics class. One area in the body can change another area since they are interconnected.

It is not unusual that this shoulder patient is often excited at first because we just demonstrated a solution that could work to fix their long-term problems by fixing the hip or other areas of tightness that caused the shoulder problem. This reaction, however, is often followed by frustration in that they had seen so many other clinicians beforehand that did not help them because they did not look in these other places. In the defense of those other clinicians, as mentioned before, most are just not trained to look beyond the shoulder for the cause of the shoulder injury. **You have to be trained to fix the system in order to fix the symptoms**.

The example of the hip above is just one example. We have 206 bones and close to 600 muscles in the body. Combine that with however many years of life you have lived, you have probably had many moments of impact and injury that have led to many key areas of tightness in multiple places in the body. Thus, I tell my staff and patients that we will see many shoulder problems in a month and year, but we will technically never see the same patient twice. Everyone has their own special presentation. You are unique.

Think back over your life. In addition to shoulder issues, have you ever had pain or problems in any other parts of your body? It does not have to be "bad enough" that you sought out medical care for it. Maybe it was just a moment or a day with pain or stiffness or weakness. Have you ever hurt your:

- Lower back?
- Neck/head?
- Elbows?
- Hands?
- Ribs?
- Hips?
- Knees?
- Feet?
- Tailbone?
- Other areas?

Any muscle in the body can hold tightness if it has been challenged at any time in your life. That area of tightness changes the alignment and motion of the tissues next to it. Changes in that one area then leads to changes in the bones, muscles, and tissues that then attach to **that** area. Before you know it, many other parts of your body are affected by the injury of that initial area of tightness. Due to a chain reaction, you could have a problem in your big toe that gives you a headache. You could have a change in your neck that leads to a foot pain. It is all connected. I have had chronic pain patients like those with a "fibromyalgia" diagnosis that thought they had twenty different problems just to find out that they really had only one or two problems that created twenty issues over a period of time. And when you identify and fix those key areas of restriction, you fix twenty problems at the same time!

You may be reading this and think, "Of course! The body is connected. One area affects another!" However, if you went to medical school, PT school, or other areas of education, you would find that this is really not how we are taught to view the body and treat injuries in our western medicine culture. When you learn about the shoulder in class, you will typically just learn a million tests and treatments just for the shoulder area itself and you will not be taught to see the larger picture at almost any of these institutions. There are a few voices out there in continuing education that have preached this for decades. I am hopeful along with the education we are doing, and with this book, that eventually everyone will learn to assess the body by **fixing the system to fix the symptoms.**

Any change to one part of your body will affect what happens to the other parts of the body. These changes could be positive or negative. Improving one area can improve other areas alongside it. Injuring one part of the body has negative consequences elsewhere. Improving that one area has positive benefits elsewhere.

Key Thought #6: You must see the tightness in the system to fix the symptoms.

CHAPTER SEVEN

SHARE THE WORKLOAD AND WORK THE POWER ZONES

There is another mechanism in which tightness in the body in one area leads to injuries elsewhere. To understand this, we go back to good old physics class. (I bet you said back in school you would never use that information in the future real world. You were wrong!) In this section, we will analyze the following equation.

Pressure = Force divided by area
$$P = F/A$$

In this equation, think of "*area*" as the total amount of parts of the body that can perform a given motion or activity. For example, in the picture below, as this heavy object is lifted, examine how many joints are being moved to perform that task. The ankles are bending. The knees and hips are bending as well. The joints are moving, and the muscles are working around them to make that happen.

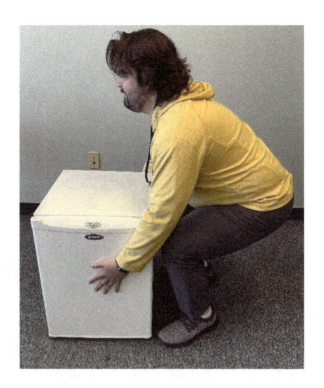

Since P=F/A, the **GREATER THE AREA** of bones and muscles you have that can take on that task, the **LESSER THE PRESSURE** will then result on each individual part.

Now let's create a scenario where this person in the picture below has really tight hips. In this scenario, the hips cannot bend as well to help with that heavy lift. So what do the knees think about that? The knees must **WORK A LOT HARDER** to make up for the work the hips did not do. Over time, the knees will get injured from the overuse. But the knee injury was not due to poor knee muscles, but rather the hip area not doing its job due to tightness.

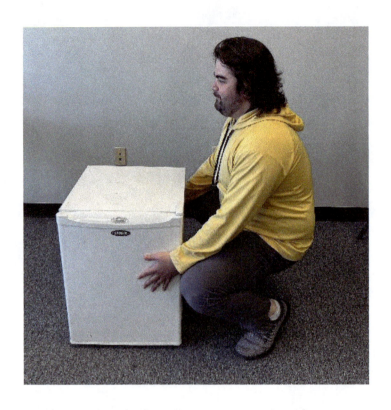

Let's now say that I have a patient with really tight hips plus really weak knees. Now they must lift up the box with mostly their spine. Since there is less area of parts of the body moving, the knees and back are not helping, there is MORE pressure and work on the spine. The spine then gets overworked, and this person now has back pain! But again, it is not the spine's fault in this example. The fault lies in the knees and hips not doing their proper jobs.

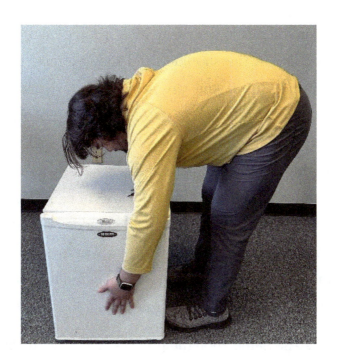

Make sense? Now let's take this example back to the shoulder. When we move and use our arms, as discussed before, we need the shoulder blade and collar bone to move as well. But the shoulder blade and collar bone will only move as well as the mid back, ribs, neck, lower back, hips, and other parts of the body allow them to move. The less the **AREA** of parts moving, the more **PRESSURE** gets on the shoulder. Eventually this leads to shoulder injury if those other parts of the body are not moving properly and doing their job to take pressure off of the work in the shoulders.

You have to **fix the system to fix the symptoms** of the shoulder pain. Lack of contribution from those other areas leads to overwork in the shoulder. It is often not the area of tightness but rather the overworked area that gets the pain. So how should treatment look if this is the case? Most people take the painful injured area like in the shoulder and they exercise the painful shoulder more! But if the problem is that the shoulder is overworked from the other parts of the body not functioning properly, all you are doing in that situation is adding EXTRA WORK to the OVERWORKED area! By overworking it even further, you just add more pain to the area of pain. Make sense? So the secret to fixing the overworked shoulder would be to do treatments that lessen the tightness and weakness of the other parts of the body so that the overworked shoulder can be more relaxed and just doing its normal role.

Using the same thought process, go back to that heavy object above that was to be lifted from the floor. Now imagine that you are the one who has to lift that item and that it weighs 250 pounds! You have the option of either trying to lift it by yourself, or you can bring in some friends to help you out on the other corners. Which choice is nicer to your body? Of course, it's easier to have friend help, right? Share the load. P=F/A. The more things that can take on work, the less the strain on the individual part.

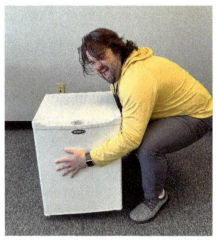

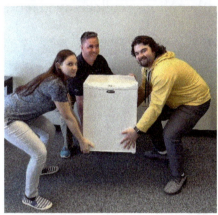

Power Zones

Taking that principle from above one step further, we realize that not all muscles and bones are made the same. I tell people that God makes some muscles and bones larger and some muscles and bones smaller. When you examine functional anatomy, you will discover that the larger muscles and bones are designed for higher force and heavier work to be put on them. The smaller muscles and bones are more for fine-tuned and more detailed tasks.

So, if you had to have some muscles and bones in particular to be healthy in such a way that a shoulder would be thankful for their assistance, you want to begin by looking at the larger areas that are better at taking on force and work. The harder the larger muscles can work, the less the shoulder has to work.

Let us go back to the example earlier of having friends help you to lift that heavy box. Now let's give you **choices** of those friends. You can either choose college-aged football linemen with

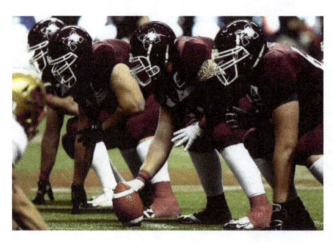

huge muscles or choose skinny eighty-year-old men to help you out with that heavy lift. Which one of those choices would be easier on **your** body? You would choose the football players, right?

These areas of larger muscles and bones that can better take on higher forces, are called the "**power zones**". You do not necessarily have to know the anatomical names for them like we do. Scan your body and ask yourself, where do you see larger muscles compared to other muscles? You might see larger muscles in your thighs, butt, calf, abdomen, and chest, for example. These are good examples of power zones.

Contrast that with the muscles around the foot, hand, neck, and other smaller muscle and bone groups that cannot take on as much force. By making sure to keep the larger parts of

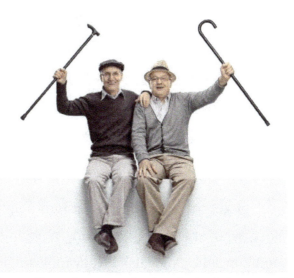

the body flexible, active, aligned properly in their joints and strong, you will reap even greater benefits to your shoulder problem than you would from improving the smaller bones and muscles. If you apply this to the equation P=F/A, having a larger **area (A)** of power zones working well will take even further **pressure (P)** off your shoulder than would the smaller areas.

Key Thought #7: Having a larger amount of body parts that can move well, especially in the power zones, leads to less strain on the shoulder and thus greater healing.

CHAPTER EIGHT

DO I NEED AN X-RAY OR MRI BEFORE I CONSIDER STARTING ANY TREATMENT PROGRAM?

I get this question about radiology a lot in the clinic from those who are calling us and inquiring about our help with shoulder pain. They ask if they have to get an X-ray or MRI first before they come to our therapy clinic. In some cases, they are concerned because the test is very expensive, and their insurance does not cover the cost. An MRI can cost thousands of dollars out of pocket. But those same people can be concerned that we NEED these tests in order to properly diagnose and treat their shoulder pains.

Like a good teacher, I typically respond by answering their question with a couple of other questions. I ask...

1. Was there any major trauma to that arm that led to this pain?
2. Can you raise your arm above the height of your shoulder to the front and side angles?

If someone had a major trauma and is not able to lift the arm above the height of the shoulder, then radiology might be helpful. X-rays will mostly show if there has been a fracture, but they will not show any tears of tendons, ligaments or muscles. MRIs are better at showing rotator cuff tears.

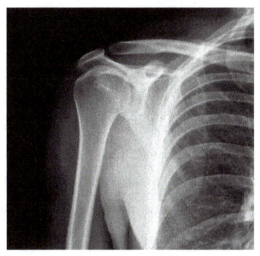

X-ray of shoulder

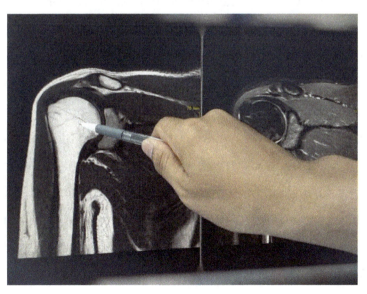

MRI of shoulder

The real question about getting extra radiology is, does that person need **surgery right now** with their shoulder problem? If the answer is maybe or yes, radiology is beneficial in the decision-making process and can help to justify such a procedure. However, let's say that a patient does not want surgery right now, or they did not have any major arm trauma, or they can raise their arm at least the height of their shoulder if not higher. If any of those situations are true, I find that radiology is usually not that beneficial to us. This is because our treatment is usually going to be conservative and the results of the radiology do not help the clinician in the design of the treatment plan.

A good clinical evaluation is typically much more helpful at identifying a plan of action for conservative treatment than radiology. By also examining not just the shoulder but also the mechanics and tight areas elsewhere in the body, a good clinician can come up with a more detailed treatment plan than you could from just radiology in cases where surgery is not yet needed or desired. Observing the mechanics of how the shoulder moves and which parts of the body are restricting that normal motion gives us more information than pictures. Especially after the age of 30, we all have some noticeable wear and tear on our shoulders that could be seen on radiology. But obviously, most of us do not have any shoulder pain or we do have minor pains that do not need surgery.

The good news is that a good clinical evaluation will also tell the therapist if radiology is appropriate as well. If someone comes to see me on day one and they have certain "red flag" tests, we will send them on ahead for that surgical consult and radiology. Thankfully, a very high percentage of the time, non-surgical conservative methods are called for at first. So that patient can save a lot of money by not getting extra, unnecessary testing and still get the shoulder better by using the appropriate conservative treatments.

Key Thought #8: Most of the time you can start a therapy program without having radiology done on the shoulder. Radiology is most helpful when there is extreme trauma or concern that a surgery is needed instead of conservative treatment.

CHAPTER NINE

THE FIVE MOST COMMON SHOULDER INJURIES

We have discussed how shoulder injuries occur when the scapula has tightness that does not allow it to "get out of the way", and the humerus then pinches in to the top of the shoulder blade bone and compresses the tissues in between. This tightness, as previously discussed, could have its origin in any other part of the body that could create this shoulder pinching. These same mechanics are basically the cause of all the five most common shoulder injuries, with some having more severity and concern than others.

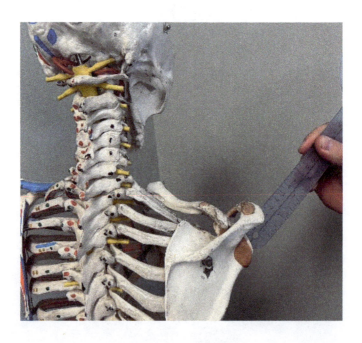

1. Shoulder impingement syndrome (the easiest one to fix)

If you must have a shoulder problem, the most desirable one to have is the **shoulder impingement**. This can be extremely painful, but compared to the other categories we will discuss, it is the easiest one to fix in the shortest amount of time. Later, I will show you my favorite four exercises for helping with shoulder pain. If you have the shoulder impingement syndrome and not one of the other four diagnoses, after performing even the first exercise on that list, you will already notice an obvious improvement with your shoulder problem.

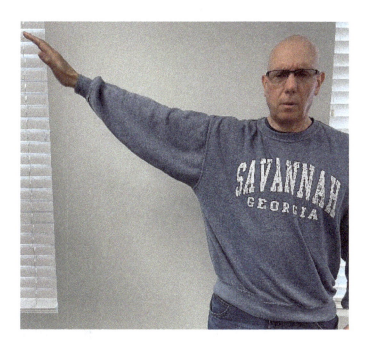

The shoulder impingement basically means this pinching of the tissues in between the two bones has now led to pain and inflammation of those tissues due to that compression. When the arm reaches to this impingement point and hits a "block", thus irritating certain tissues like the supraspinatus tendon, the arm bone can then also shift forward and irritate the biceps tendon. Because these tendons are often irritated, many have called this problem "tendinitis" in the past. Tendinitis is one kind of a correct diagnosis in this case of impingement.

However, there is also a bursa in this area called the subacromial bursa that gets compressed in this impingement problem as well. Think of a bursa as an empty balloon of tissue that God puts in certain parts of our body to help to decrease friction of muscles and tendons rubbing near bones. But if one of these bursae gets compressed and irritated enough, it fills up with fluid and gets inflamed. Irritation of this bursa has led many to call this diagnosis "bursitis" in the past, which is also correct due to the inflamed bursa. There are also ligaments that can get squished in this impingement.

Because all these tissues are typically pinched together at the same time, most clinicians do not use words like "tendinitis" or "bursitis" as much these days. Instead, we clump all of those problems together and call this injury the "impingement syndrome".

Most impingement patients will begin to get relief on the first day of treatment. Typical treatment time to fully recover from an impingement and clean up all the tight mechanics that caused the shoulder problem is usually close to around five weeks. Obviously, some shoulder cases could be easier, and some could be more challenging depending on the time, depth, and complexity of the presentation.

2. Partial rotator cuff tear

Tears of the rotator cuff tendons and other surrounding tissues can happen with trauma. But most of the time, as mentioned previously, the tears happen because of repetitive actions with poor mechanics that leads to longer term impingement. In other words, if you have an impingement and you do not properly treat the shoulder AND the tight mechanics from the rest of the body that caused that impingement, you will likely have a partial rotator cuff tear eventually.

The good news is that the partial tear is still typically treated with conservative methods like therapy and not surgery yet. The same mechanical issues that cause the impingement syndrome are what causes the partial tear, so the treatments are very similar. Typically, the partial tear patient will also make some improvements that can be measured even on a first day in therapy or with one of the exercises I will show later in the book. But the improvements will be smaller than with the impingement patient.

The bad news is that the time to clean up a partial tear in therapy is usually a couple more weeks than the impingement. The risk level is also higher in this category that a little more time with this problem or a fall or trauma on that arm could easily change someone from a partial tear to the next category.

3. Complete "full thickness" rotator cuff tear

At this level, typically you are not able to raise your arm to the height of your shoulder. Over the years, we have been able to improve the mechanics of the functionality of someone's spine, neck, shoulder blade, and other parts of the body to where they can function more comfortably with this complete tear problem. But if you desire to have full normal pain free function of the arm again, this is where surgery is typically needed. A full rotator cuff procedure also brings challenges in recovery. Typically, you must leave the arm in an immobilizing sling for weeks and very slowly and carefully start to regain motion and strength back with challenging and uncomfortable therapy treatments.

We are thankful that such rotator cuff surgeries exist, but life would have been so much easier, and the recovery would have been so much quicker and less painful had that person sought out care when in the previous two easier categories of the impingement or partial tear. It is usually around six months before the surgically repaired shoulder feels back to full normal function again.

There are times when the first surgery was not enough, and further surgeries are needed later. In my experience, patients often wonder if they had a "bad surgeon" or flawed therapy that led to such an undesired outcome. I find the main reason why a surgery would "fail" and require additional procedures is not that the surgeon did a poor performance but rather once again that the tightness in the system discussed earlier was never addressed. The mechanics of the pinching are still omnipresent in the form of tightness in the rest of the body. Then as time goes along, the same faulty mechanics lead to more impingement and then more tears and more future procedures. Once again, you have to **fix the system to fix the symptoms.**

4. Adhesive Capsulitis/"The Frozen Shoulder"

You might be tempted to think that the surgery with the complete tear is the worst-case scenario. If it was my shoulder, this fourth category is possibly even worse than the surgical one. The good news with the surgical scenario is that usually you feel a lot better after six months. In this next category, known as adhesive capsulitis, or slang as the "frozen shoulder", it can take 1.5 to 2 years to get your normal motion and function back in the shoulder. With good therapy and treatment, the time is certainly lessened. In my experience with treating all kinds of different muscle and joint injuries over the years, this frozen shoulder is the absolute slowest and patience-challenging diagnosis to treat of all of the different orthopedic problems we see from any part of the body.

Basically, in a frozen shoulder, you will see every muscle in the neighborhood of the shoulder go into "lockdown" mode. This problem may or may not have pain associated with it. But you will see major difficulties in moving that arm in almost any direction, making use of the arm extremely challenging to do day-to-day needs and simple activities.

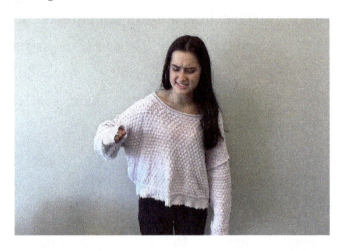

What causes the frozen shoulder to occur as compared to the previous diagnoses? The truth is that after years of many people examining that question, we are still not exactly sure what leads to adhesive capsulitis. It is almost as if the brain senses that there is something so sinister going on in that joint, that it locks down the muscles to restrict the shoulder from moving. Then after two years of inactivity, if there has been some healing, the muscles can then relax and allow motion to begin again in the arm. If you research looking for causes of frozen shoulder, you may see correlations with this problem can occur tied to these issues below:

- Trauma
- Stroke
- Continued stress on a Rotator Cuff tear
- Poor recovery from shoulder surgery

- Circulatory medical issues like diabetes or heart disease
- Hormonal issues like thyroid deficiencies or overactivity
- More serious diseases like tuberculosis
- Neurological and brain issues such as Parkinson's
- And there are more....

The most common reason why I see a frozen shoulder in the clinic still ties back to those same tight bodily restrictions leading to impingement, then tears, and then to this level where the body goes in to "lockdown" mode to protect itself. Treatment again is **very slow and very agonizing**. When I diagnose someone with adhesive capsulitis, I usually pause and shake their hand and ask, "Do you like me alright so far? Because we are going to know each other for a **LONG** time."

5. Shoulder instability

The last category lies with those who have difficulty keeping the humerus in the socket of the shoulder blade. When the arm with instability is moved, instead of remaining properly in the socket, the head of the humerus wants to roll to the edges and in some cases even beyond the boundary of the cup.

When the arm has a brief moment where it goes out of socket, but then returns back into position, this is called a **subluxation**. When the arm stays out of socket, it is called a **dislocation**. Treatment includes putting the humerus back in to position if needed, but then performing techniques that promote a more stable environment for the future.

This is where I find that most clinicians are taught improperly on how to create that stability. Traditional protocol calls for a variety of "rotator cuff exercises" to be performed on the loose shoulder to try to increase their ability to be stronger at keeping the arm in the socket. We are taught that the instability of the shoulder comes from ligaments that are too loose. Traditional treatment thought says that since it is not possible to contract ligaments to get them stronger and tighter, one must accept the ligamentous instability and try to make up for that laxity with more efficient shoulder muscles.

Over the years, we have found a significantly better approach at shoulder stability. The answer still lies in looking again at **the system** and not just the **symptom**. We have found that you can still have a stable shoulder with loose ligaments if the anatomy of the other parts of the body that move with the shoulder are also similarly very flexible. As discussed, when you move your arm, your shoulder blade, clavicle, spine, ribs, pelvic, and hip areas should be moving along with the arm. I have found that pretty much 100% of my "loose" shoulder patients that can sublux and dislocate their arm happen to also have a quite tight set of bones and muscles adjacent to the arm. This is especially seen in the mid back (thoracic) and hip areas. When you focus on loosening up the tight areas in the system, the shoulder blade is then free to move easily with the arm. Thus the socket moves with the humerus and creates a functionally more stable shoulder.

Key Thought #9: Barring a trauma, tightness in the system is what causes the five different types of shoulder injury. The five different shoulder injuries are: impingement, partial rotator cuff tear, full rotator cuff tear, adhesive capsulitis, and instability.

CHAPTER TEN

COMMON TREATMENT OPTIONS OUTSIDE OF THERAPY

Most of the time, when someone first hurts their shoulder, as mentioned in previous chapters, their first choices of treatment are ignoring it, resting it, and trying over the counter medications to help with the pain and inflammation. If these steps do not resolve the issue, the common next step is to go to see their primary care doctor. There are definitely great primary care doctors out there that are champions at presenting all of the different choices for treatment. These are the doctors that are best helping their patients to come to an informed option for fixing the shoulder problem.

However, I have found a very large percentage of primary care doctors tend to go through some form of the protocol below which is less than ideal in my opinion.

First step by primary care MDs: try prescription medications.

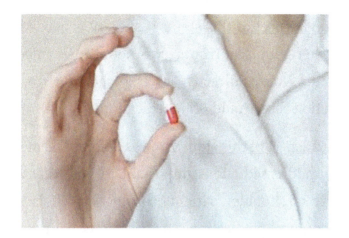

Good aspect of this step: Stronger anti-inflammatories can help cut down the inflammation better than over the counter medications.

Bad aspect of this step: Drugging the shoulder does nothing to change the mechanics of what causes most shoulder problems to occur. If you do not fix the mechanics, the shoulder problems will continue and usually get worse over time. Also, prescription medications bring with them at times unwanted side effects.

Second step by primary care MDs: Refer to an orthopedic surgeon.

Orthopedic doctors primarily do two forms of treatment that most primary care doctors do not perform for shoulder problems:

1. Injections (typically cortisone or some steroid)
2. Surgery

<u>Good aspect of this step</u>: If surgery is needed, they have come to the right place. If surgery is not needed, injections often still do act more directly at the shoulder to cut down inflammation than would oral medications.

<u>Bad aspect of this step</u>: Same as before. The mechanics are not being addressed. It is important to note that a very high percentage of shoulder patients can be very effectively treated without surgery, medications, or injections. So this orthopedic visit becomes an unnecessary step if that is the case.

Some doctors also rarely suggest or try:

- Physical therapy
- Chiropractic treatment
- Massage therapy
- Acupuncture
- Personal training in a gym or outside group
- Nutritional counseling
- Prayer
- And other options...

Obviously, each of these choices can have their own set of benefits and limitations.

So what do we wish most people and primary care doctors would do first when shoulder pain occurs?

The question here might be, "Who is in the best position to be the gatekeeper for problems such as shoulder pain?" The answer would have to be a clinician who specializes in muscle and joint biomechanics, but who also has the skill to screen out the "red flag" test scenarios to know if a surgical consult is appropriate. We would say that physical therapists are the best suited to be these initial gatekeepers. I typically get close to an hour with patients on their first session to conduct a thorough examination, begin some treatment, and then make an appropriate plan for moving forward.

A good doctor may spend a maximum of 10 minutes unless the patient is a surgical case. This is not their fault. Their schedule dictates this routine. Since most of the time surgery is not needed in shoulder pain, and more conservative treatment is called for, the therapist would be more well-suited to begin an appropriate conservative treatment plan on day one than would the doctor. A good therapist would also screen to see if radiology or treatment with other professionals is deemed appropriate.

Key Thought #10: The traditional flow of treatment options in medicine for shoulder pain has flaws. It is best to start with a movement specialist like a PT who can screen and send to others as needed, or choose to start treatment to correct the mechanical problem without unnecessary surgeries or medications.

CHAPTER ELEVEN

WHY TRADITIONAL EXERCISE CAN MAKE YOU WORSE

The information I am getting ready to share is probably going to stress out a certain number of you. This is especially true for those who have enjoyed spending countless hours in gyms for a decent percentage of their lives. So be prepared to handle this next statement...

When you have mechanics that cause shoulder problems, traditional strengthening and stretching exercises will typically cause you more HARM than good. As such, these exercises should be avoided.

There... I said it. And yes... I am a physical therapist. If I went back to physical therapy school tomorrow (instead of *what feels like* way back in the 1800s when I was in school), the professors there would be shocked that I made my statement above. Those professors are still most likely teaching that in order to decrease pain, increase range of motion, and increase strength and function, you have to take the "bad" injured arm and stretch it and work the muscles with strengthening exercises. In other words, take the injured, restricted arm and force it to move through its limitations to get to the goal.

Breaking it down... why would I make this bold statement? First of all, the majority of clinicians have used this treatment strategy in the clinic for many years. Shoulder patients come into the physical therapy sessions with a tight and painful arm. Those clinicians either assist that patient to stretch that injured arm or they make that patient stretch it themselves. They give that patient dumbbells, therabands, and other tools to work on strengthening for that injured arm. Back in the 1980s and 1990s, the intensity of this work would often be in the "No Pain, No Gain" category. Patients would then often walk out of the sessions feeling really sore and painful in their arms, but the clinician would just chalk it up to the "It's good for you. It's how it is done" category. Then we would pray the inflammation and pain would calm down enough between sessions so the next time we could do it all over again.

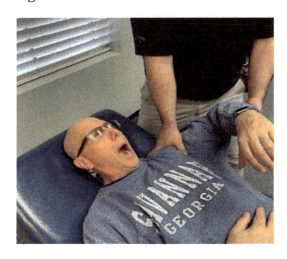

After the 1990s, clinicians began to realize the flaws in those thoughts. However, adjustments were mostly made in intensity, where the stretching and exercises would be done to less painful levels, but otherwise would look similar in form to prior decades.

Why does this strategy have such a decent chance at failure? To understand this, reflect back on previous chapters where we discussed how the tightness in the system leads the humerus bone to "pinch" into the roof of the shoulder blade in these injuries. This tightness again could be from the neck, mid back, lower back, hips, or other areas. Shoulder injuries would occur when someone would try to move that arm, but since the muscles and bones next to the arm were not moving properly due to that systemic tightness, the arm would pinch those rotator cuff tendons, ligaments, bursae, etc. When one goes to "stretch the injured arm" in sessions, basically they are just further forcing the humerus into this pinch. Of course, this leads to more pain, inflammation, and injury. Therefore, what is called "treatment" is really just forcing the arm into the injury zone itself.

What about strengthening exercises? They could be even worse than stretching for two reasons. First, you are adding more force into the same pinch that you were doing with the prior stretching. Second, when you contract the muscles of the "bad arm," that contraction creates a shortening of that muscle tissue on that injured arm side. This shortening causes a "pulling" effect on the muscles to which they attach. For example, if the injured arm is the right shoulder, if you contract to try to strengthen the right arm itself, those right-sided muscles will pull the right neck, right mid back, right lower back, and other areas MORE to the RIGHT!

Think of it like the picture below where you have a right shoulder problem. In the first picture, when the arm is at rest, the tightness from the injury is pulling those muscles and bones more towards the right shoulder. Working strengthening exercises on the right arm would then pull those bones and muscles further to the right, like we see the pulling of the shirt in the second picture.

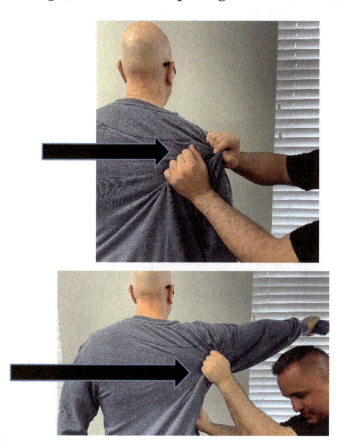

In this example, the tight right neck and spinal muscles were causing the right shoulder problem. Now the right arm exercises are pulling the alignments and tensions of these areas FURTHER out of balance to the right side. This essentially not only strains the shoulder itself, but also worsens the other areas of the neck and spine that are out of balance to the right that were causing the problem in the first place!

Make sense?

So, then, what is the next question you need to ask? Are there any exercises then that are helpful to healing these types of injuries? Exercises that not only would help fix the shoulder problem itself, but that also could correct those neck, spine and other muscles and joints that caused the problem in the first place.

The answer, ABSOLUTELY HECK YEAH!

Key Thought #11: Traditional shoulder stretching and strengthening exercises can add to the injury more than help heal the injury. In order to heal with exercise, you must consider other options.

CHAPTER TWELVE

HOW TO KNOW IF TREATMENT IS WORKING –

THE SECRET OF "TREAT"

When you are a kid and get sick, you learn you need to "trust your doctor." This is a good thing. Your doctor has had many years of schooling and experience to assist in helping you get healthy again. However, I have found that full and unquestioning trust in medical professionals of all types can have serious flaws. I refer to this flaw as the "white coat syndrome." This is when a patient basically blindly trusts their doctor, therapist, or other specialist, no matter what the results are showing.

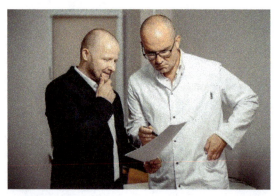

For example, just a few weeks ago, a patient asked me, "What do you think of me still seeing my chiropractor?" I told her that there are many amazing chiropractors and many poor ones that are crooks to stay away from. I told her I feel that way also about therapists, doctors, and other clinicians. But in general, I like chiropractors and I share patients with them all the time with a successful teamwork that leads to a successful outcome. However, I told this lady I needed to follow up her question with some questions of my own:

- "How long have you been seeing this chiropractor?"
- "How do you feel after your sessions?"
- "If you feel better after the sessions, how long does the relief last?"
- "Over the period of time that you have been seeing this chiropractor, have you made progress in a way in which you are satisfied?"

The answers were that this lady had been seeing the chiropractor every month for around 20 years. Every time she went, she would leave feeling better. The relief would typically last a day or two before returning to baseline. And over the last two decades, in general, the problem has had a net worsening.

How did I answer her question about what I thought about her seeing her chiropractor? I told her that her answers to my questions were the answer to her question! Basically, her chiropractic sessions were helpful, as evidenced by the two day relief period. But they were not sufficient enough to maintain progress and head her toward a solid, long-term positive and healing solution. Over time, the net result was not progressing and actually worsening.

I had another patient who recently came to our therapy clinic after having been treated at another PT clinic for twice a week for close to a year for his shoulder problem. This guy never left a single one of his previous therapy sessions feeling any better and would usually feel worse after those treatments were performed. Over time, he continued to get worse. So, what was I thinking? First, why did he keep going there for so long if he knew it wasn't working?

The answer is that he just **assumed** that he was doing what he was supposed to do. He was not aware of any other options, he wanted to do something for his pain and he did not want surgery or medications. The clinician treating him also never admitted that the treatments were not working and that other options should be explored. So he just kept going to that PT until someone else had suggested to him giving our different type of therapy a try.

Basically, **the result is the result**. I tell people all the time to not just trust anything I say to them just because I said it. I have come up with some brilliant ideas over the years that would totally fail and not work on a given specific patient. In contrast, I have come up with some of the weirdest and stupidest ideas you could ever imagine that would actually work really well with a given patient!

The most important thing is to always have some form of **measurable goal**. If the treatment is working, we should see it working. The progress should be measurable. Progress could take the form of less pain, greater motion, greater strength, functional improvement, etc. We want to measure a "better." At first those gains may be milder and shorter term. But we should see, over time, those results gaining in amplitude and sustainability. Any action that leads to a positive result should be seen as a helper and should be continued. Any action that leads to a no change or a worsening result, we should recognize as such and not continue to perform that task in the same manner as before as we move forward.

My first years as a therapist, I worked at a great clinic in Knoxville, Tennessee. They used a tool called FOTO (Focus on Therapeutic Outcomes) that would measure the outcomes of how well a patient would improve with therapy. The way this worked is that the patient would answer questions on a computer on the first and last sessions. Then data would be entered on the last session showing how many times they attended, the total treatment cost, etc. The input would be made into statistical data that could be tracked and used to compare therapists to each other in the company, and to others all over the country to see how each clinician stacked up against each other and national norms.

When I was fresh out of school, I knew I was new. I did not hide the fact that I had a lot to learn. One of the reasons I chose to work where I did was that I liked how there were a lot more experienced and smarter therapists that I could learn from. They also had a fantastic continuing educational program in place. And believe me, I did learn a lot from them. However, to my surprise, when these FOTO statistics would be released, I always, always ranked right at or near the top of outcomes when compared to other therapists in both the company and around the country. I was getting patients better relief and better gains in less time and less cost than the more experienced clinicians. This confused me and even embarrassed me a bit because I knew my knowledge base and experience was so much less than theirs.

Looking back on it, how do I believe that I achieved that kind of measurable success in patient outcomes? The answer is actually pretty simple. When I was working there, even early on, it became obvious to me that certain therapists in the company had found their pet, favorite forms of treatment. Each PT was different in what types of treatments they performed, but they would do those same favorite treatments with every patient over and over and over again. If a patient came for twenty sessions with a certain therapist, they would often get the exact same treatment on every session. If the treatment worked and they got better, that was great. But if the treatment was not working, that poor result would typically not change the treatment strategy at all. The same therapist would continue that same treatment for 10, 20, 30 or more sessions basically until that patient would eventually quit and return to their doctor with a failed outcome.

Having a little more humility, I would tell myself that I did not know what each patient specifically needed for their best treatments. I knew that I had several treatment options to choose from that I had learned in school and from continuing education after graduation. I started by conducting the initial evaluation and tried the first treatment choice that I thought was best based on the diagnosis and presentation. If that first option was working, I would continue that path. However, if the first treatment option did not show adequate progress, then I would try some alteration of the first treatment or some other completely different option. The search would continue, unique to each patient, until I would find that one recipe that was working individually for that person. To me, then and now, each patient was like their own puzzle for me to solve that needed their own specific answer.

So, what's the moral of the story? **The number one friend of any patient or clinician who wants to get better the fastest way possible should be my TREAT philosophy below.** There should always be measurements taken. Always. The results should then dictate the next actions, not just the preference of the clinician or patient. TREAT is an anagram for the process below:

T: **TEST** the problem in a measurable way. Then try the initial treatment.

R: **RETEST** the same measure after the first treatment is completed.

E: **EXAMINE** the result of the retest. (Better? Worse? No change?)

A: **APPLY** the result into the next action. If the treatment helped, do more of what helped. If it did not, make an adjustment and try something new.

T: **TEST**, treat, and retest again, over and over. This keeps going on until you get to the desired result.

The results dictate the actions. Do not get stuck in just doing what you think is right. Do what is measurably working. Keep it simple.

Key Thought #12: Apply the principles of "TREAT," with constant testing, retesting, and making adjustments as needed in order to get to the desired result in the fastest way possible.

CHAPTER THIRTEEN

INTRODUCTION TO TMR (TOTAL MOTION RELEASE) – A BETTER OPTION

I moved back home to Raleigh, North Carolina, from Knoxville, Tennessee around 2002. At that time, I had learned a lot already from my prior years about how to be an effective physical therapist and in the treatment of bodily pains, including shoulder issues. But there were still some problems that I had never figured out how to solve. I list some of them below.

1. Of all the techniques I had ever learned, **nothing had ever helped me personally** with my own chronic pains of around 20 years! Absolutely nothing. I had several issues with back pain, sciatica issues, severe tail bone pain to where I was unable to sit, foot pain (plantar fasciitis), right knee problems, vertigo, and other issues. If you ever meet another physical therapist, you will find that most of us get in this profession because we ourselves are physically screwed up specimens! I had tried every type of treatment I saw out there with little to zero success. It was very deflating. Can you relate to how I felt back then?

2. I recognized the power of the whole-body connection, but there were very few experts in continuing education that could help teach us how to refine those connections into an effective tool on how to properly fix pains. How do we put it all together? I went to a course in 2000 by a therapist named Gary Gray. His course was 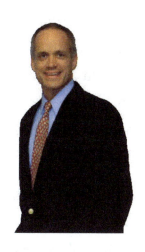 called "Chain Reaction, Explosion!" It was the first voice I had heard that was making these connections scientific in a way that was also common sense and measurable. This course completely changed how I saw the body move, how it gets injuries, and how it should heal. But Gary's voice and these concepts were unfortunately the exception and not the rule in therapy and the medical profession. So it was difficult to take those thoughts further than the basic concepts.

3. The "working into the painful restriction" philosophy never fully made sense to me, but I had never really known how to explore other possibilities. So, I just did what the majority typically did in our profession. This is where the Lord led me to pack up and leave a very secure job situation in Tennessee and come to work for a new boss at Total Motion Physical Therapy in Raleigh. His name was Tom Dalonzo-Baker.

At first meeting, I knew that Tom was an interesting bird. I felt from him a mixture of feelings where I thought he was either crazy, brilliant, or a bit of both. The idea of working for him was interesting to me but also made me nervous. I knew he had a different set of skills and thought processes that I had not yet considered. The idea of learning and trying something new sounded attractive enough to the point where I took my wife and three children and moved back to Raleigh where I had grown up.

Tom saw the world and how the body heals in ways that most people did not, and most clinicians did not learn in traditional education. Despite all our personality and other differences, what I liked about Tom early on was also how we were alike. This especially included his desire to always have continual improvement, an impatience with the status quo, his recognition of the full body mechanics, and his usage of the test and retest (what I later refined into Chip's TREAT steps in Chapter 12) with how he took care of his patients. He also shared my thoughts as I mentioned above that the result is the result and that should dictate one's choices. If an action is performed that is increasing pain, that treatment choice is usually not good. Therefore, traditional treatments that force the arm in to increased pain are forcing the body into places that the body is telling us that it does not want to do! And those choices should be avoided. By contrast, treatments that lead to improvements are to be studied, refined, celebrated, and repeated.

After I began working with him, I was also intrigued by another desire that was driving Tom forward as his primary life and professional goal. Tom wanted to create something completely new not only for physical therapy, but also for health care in general. A tool where any person could learn how to become their own clinician and fix their own pains. We could become that clinic that could "teach a man to fish and feed him for life instead of just giving a man a fish and feeding him for a day", to use that famous metaphor.

Back in 2002, most of our therapy at Total Motion PT was a manual therapy, "hands-on" based model. I had one type of hands-on training based out of Canada and Tom's training was more based on what is called myofascial release and strain-counterstrain principles. Early on in that first year of working with Tom, he began to make interesting observations such as when the body was placed into more positions of tissue comfort and softness, the manual therapy treatments themselves were more effective and easier to perform. Furthermore, when looking for those "softer" positions, he noticed that those nice comfy positions often had an opposing tight and strained option in the opposite direction. We later called these opposing positions the "good side" and the "bad side."

The next step was the realization that these working toward the "good side" treatment options were not only effective for the hands-on treatments, but they also had applications into exercises the patient could perform themselves. If you find a motion in the body where you move in one direction and you feel comfort, but in the opposite direction you feel tightness and strain, when you exercised more into the direction of the comfort, the patient would feel a lot better. Actually, they would feel a lot, lot better! This was fascinating to us. Over time, we realized that doing exercises in this manner were even giving us better results than the performance of our hands on treatments. Which is great, because the patient then has the power to "fix themselves!"

I will not bore you with the details of what then occurred over the next following months and couple of years. The truth is that we tried many options that did not work and others that worked quite well. Over time, applying this knowledge, we were able to create and refine a tool on how to fix muscle and bone pains. Thomas Edison once was asked by a reporter after he invented the light bulb what it was like to fail so many times along the way to his famous invention. I will paraphrase Mr. Edison but his answer was that he never did fail 1000 times, but rather he was on a 1000 step journey to get to the proper final answer. Tom, myself, and our clinic went on this similar Edison-like journey of creation for this tool. Along the way, something amazingly beautiful was constructed. Tom patented the flowchart of actions of this tool and named it after our clinic, calling it **Total Motion Release, or TMR for short.** A few years later, Tom sold the clinic to myself and my co-owner, Deanna Merritt. Tom continued to teach TMR all over the country and now internationally. Several thousand other clinicians use TMR with their patients as a result.

TMR Key Principle: Work to the Good Side, "Untwist the towel"

We will show a few examples in the next chapter that will help illustrate these principles of "work to the good" even further. For now, visualize a spine that is out of alignment rotated more to one side. When this happens, some muscles will be tightened on one side and some muscles will be lengthened on the other side. Some of the bones of the spine will also rub against each other, leading to tightness, decreased ability to move, and eventually pain. Visualize this concept in this spine with scoliosis below.

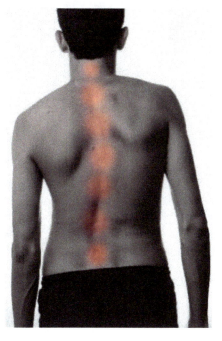

So how could a clinician do a test that shows that problem spine being rotated to one specific side without using any fancy radiology? And how could patients do that test to themselves?

And then, how could the result of that test also help one treat that problem?

First of all, imagine this towel in my hand in the picture below to be a metaphor of my spine being in a happy well aligned state with relaxed muscles.

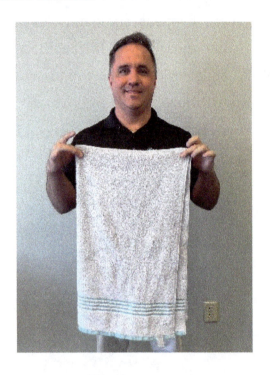

Now imagine that I got in a car accident that hit me on the left side and pushed my spine to rotate to the right. I will illustrate this also below by twisting my towel to the right like the spine was rotated that way.

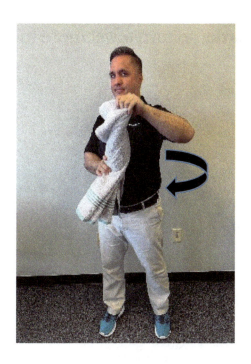

If my towel is already twisted to the right, it will make it more difficult to twist it **further** to the right, correct? However, if I wanted to twist the towel to the left, there would be more motion available on that left side. Make sense?

Harder to turn towel more to right

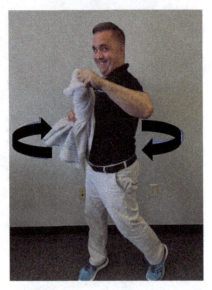

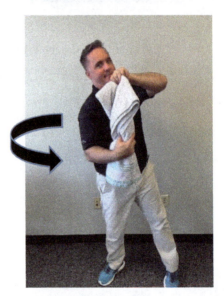

Easier to turn towel more to left

Similarly, if I sit in a chair and test my body's ability to twist my spine to the left and twist my spine to the right, I can get a good idea if my spine is in a good alignment or not by seeing if one side is harder to move than the other. If I am very flexible and symmetrical turning left and right equally, it is a good sign that my spine is in a good place. I define "good place" as bones are in a good neutral and well aligned position and the muscles around those bones are also healthy and relaxed.

However, if one side of my twist test feels more strained, tight, has less range of motion, or just in general feels harder to turn more than the other, that is a good sign that the spine is out of balance to that more restricted side.

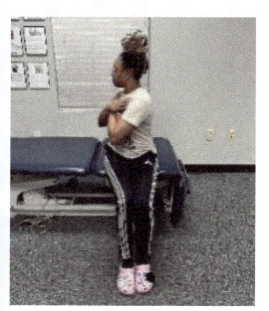 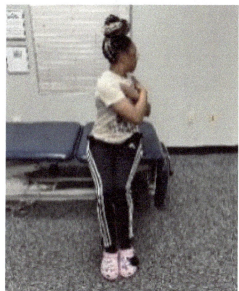

These twists look healthy symmetrical

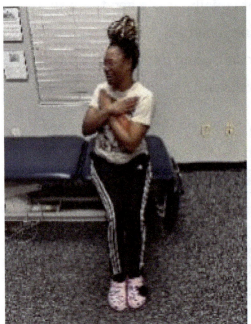 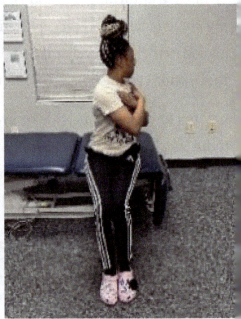

These twists look out of balance, worse to the right side

So, if the "bad side" is turning more to the right as in the picture above, this typically means the spine is aligned poorly in that right-sided direction and the muscles have also adapted to that position.

Once you know this information, how could that help you to treat that problem? You **could** try to treat the spine with exercise by turning more to the right, in the same direction as the painful restriction. But if you choose that option, basically you would take a "turned right" spine and just be turning it more to the right and into the injury! This often creates more pain and more limitation by pushing the problem more out of balance. Turning right on a spine that is already turned right is often a failed choice.

However, if I was to twist to the opposite direction, like with the towel in the example above to the left, I could possibly return that spine back to its normal position and alignment.

In the clinic, we like to test out the body, comparing motions to the left to motions on the right. This action of testing is done not only on the spine, but also the upper and lower body as well. When "imbalances" are noted where one side is more restricted to the other, we find it is more successful to exercise and work in the direction of the "good side" with the more comfortable and larger motion. This is done to restore the balance back to the body's system.

If at a later date you repeat that same test, like the body twist in the example above, and there is good symmetry at that time, you would then exercise both directions to keep that healthy balanced status. But otherwise, we are recommending working just to the one side, the one with the better motion, as long as you see those imbalances in testing.

The Secret is Balance

Basically, the key to muscle and joint health and keeping pains in the shoulder away is to have BALANCE in the system. Balance in this case we define as bones that are aligned in their proper position with muscles and other tissues in their proper lengths, positions, and tensions, etc.

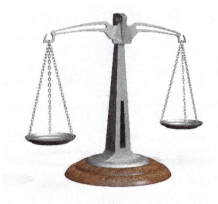

If I took you back to high school math for a moment, remember how we would graph on the x/y/z coordinate plane?

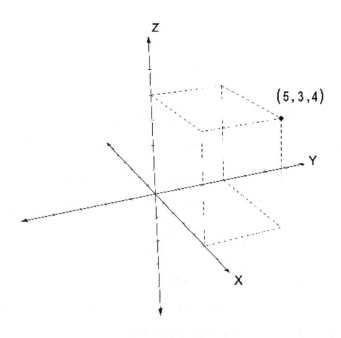

If we divide our bodies up into halves using these types of graphing lines in that graph above, you will see that we have different ways we could "slice" the body into halves. In the pictures below, observe how we can divide the body using the black line. We can have a left side and right side of our body in one "slice". We can have a front and back side of our body in another division. We can also have halves that break us up into the upper body and lower body. If you got creative, you could also come up with some fancy diagonals as well.

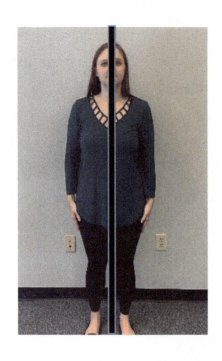
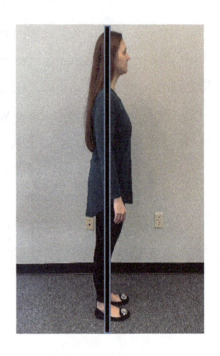

Left and Right Halves of Body

Front and Back Halves of Body

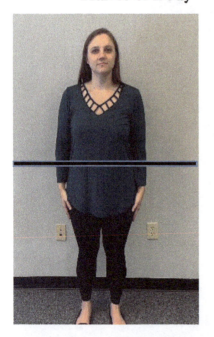

Upper and Lower Halves of Body

When any part of our body has moments of impact, those tissues tighten up in that area of impact to protect the injury. This tightness then has a "pulling effect" on the muscles and bones around it. That pulling can create a force that goes toward that one side of injury. For example, imagine someone falling really hard on their right hip.

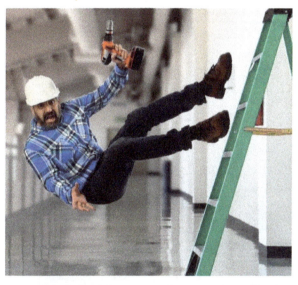

As a result of that impact, the surrounding muscles and bones will be pulled more to that right hip and away from the left hip. These forceful impacts could create also a pull with a force of upward or downward and also a pull that could be forward or backward tied to the rest of the body. The injury leads to tight pulls that draw attention towards that right hip. These tight pulls create these imbalances that I discussed earlier.

How do you correct those imbalances in the bones and muscles? If your body was pulled out of balance to the right as seen in the shirt in the picture below, you would have to pull those tissues back to the left to bring them in to balance as demonstrated with the arrow. If they were pulled upward and backward, you would have to pull downward and forward in order to get those tissues back in to balance again. It all depends on the injury. Each person has a unique history. Make sense? Now imagine that this person had had many moments of impact and injury over the years! There would be all kinds of painfully tight "pulling" going on!

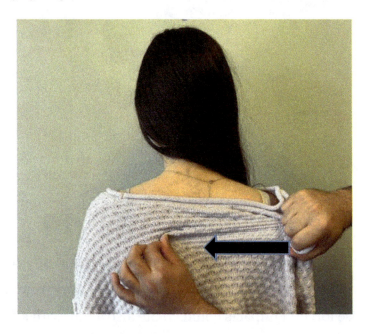

Think about how old you are. I apologize if that is a stressful thought. How many moments of impact have you had in different parts of your body over all the years in your life? Maybe you were in a car accident as a teenager. Sprained an ankle playing ball. Hurt your neck working on the computer. Injured your back working in the yard. There are many moments, correct?

Each of these moments creates an imprint of tightness on your system. Over the years, with many of these areas pulling on each other, eventually these tight tissues can start to hit certain nerves and cause our pains. Are we really more likely to have pains in the shoulder as we get older just because we are getting older itself? Or is it really from the fact that we have been alive for more years and that time allows for more moments of impact that over time tighten tissues on to our nerves? That is why you can have a pretty messed up body in a 20-year-old and a pretty decently healthy body in a 90-year-old, depending on how many impact moments have occurred.

The good news is that we do not have to be limited by our birthdays. I had around twenty years of pain that were mostly present in my younger years. I have been essentially pain free since 2004. I have less pain at fifty than I had at twenty. If you identify the areas that are out of balance and you know how to address them, you can achieve muscle and bone health, allowing you to do what you want to do without pain.

Spirit and mind balance

Another key area to keep in balance that goes even beyond our muscles and bones relates to how the body, mind, and spirit all affect each other. The more stressed we are, the more likely we are to have shoulder pain. The more shoulder pain we possess, the more likely we are to be stressed due to not enjoying life. So, we must find that balance also in our mind and spirit as well.

Is this a category that you feel out of balance in? Do you find yourself feeling constantly stressed? Do you wake up dreading the events ahead? Do you wonder why you are here on this earth and what is the purpose of your day? Do you focus more on the negative aspects of your life and have a hard time seeing the positive? Do you struggle with harboring grudges or resentment and not forgiving those who have caused you some harm in your past, like parents, spouses, friends, coworkers, or others? Do you struggle with relationships with those close to you and find loving and communicating with them to be straining?

If you answered yes to any of those questions, your mind and spirit being out of balance may be a bigger source of your pain than even just your muscles and bones themselves. I had a patient recently for whom I felt this was the case. The "home exercise" I gave to her on one session for her pains was not even physical exercise, but I told her to go home and write on a piece of paper five things she was thankful for in her life. And she should bring that sheet back with her on the next session. This was very challenging for her to do. In fact it was so challenging that I had to keep giving her that assignment over several sessions until she finally got her "five".

In my life, I have been blessed with a wonderful wife, five children, parents, family, and friends that help to keep me in balance. My wife, Nancy, is the most amazing person I have ever known, my favorite person in the world, and I am so blessed to have her in my life. When she sees me "losing my balance," she helps me to come back to center. If she sees others contributing to pull me out of balance, she will defend me like a tiger and help to protect my spirit this way as well.

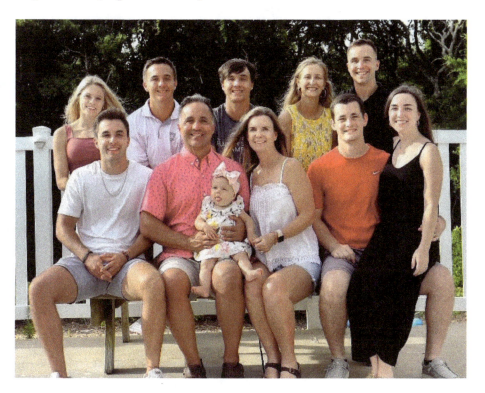

Even more important in this spiritual balance than just my relationships with these people above, is my relationship with God. Having the Lord Jesus in my life is how I can deal with the challenges from day-to-day in a more loving and peaceful manner. The purpose of my life is to give glory to Him in all my thoughts, words and deeds, and to point others in His direction as well. That relationship with the Lord is not only about having eternal security of knowing I will one day be in heaven without any of these "pains," but also how to live life itself the way it is meant to be lived. I would encourage anyone reading this book who does not understand this spiritual balance to pursue Jesus in any manner right away. My favorite Bible verse, Proverbs 3: 5-6 is illustrated on the cup below.

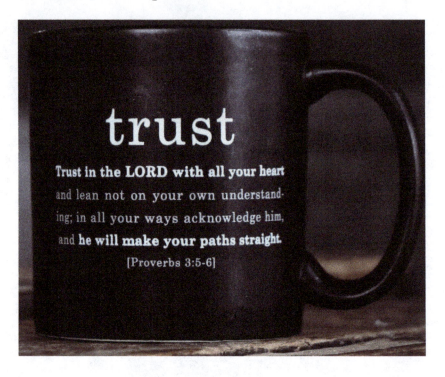

Nutritional/ Hormonal Balance

In addition to mind, body, and spiritual balance, one of the fastest advancing technologies we are seeing in treatment for bodily pains lie in our understanding of how much food and hormones influence our pains for the positive or negative. For the sake of this book, I will not go into great detail here about nutrition. However it is very possible that pain in the shoulder and body on a given person could be primarily due to poor eating habits, food allergies, or hormonal imbalances. A good way of testing out this theory is to examine how your pain is when you eat certain foods on some weeks compared to certain foods on other weeks. Can you tell a difference in your pain? Or with hormonal influences, let's say with a female, does the pain feel different at certain times of the month over other times of the month? If you see these types of patterns, it would be wise to seek out professional help with those issues to try to keep your body as healthy as possible and keep away your pains.

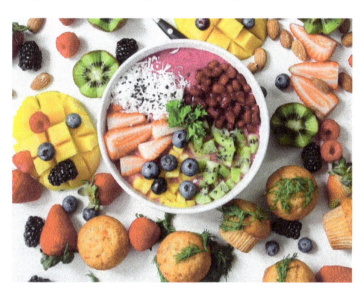

Key Thought #13: A balanced and well aligned system is healthier than one that is out of balance. Test the body by comparing motion to the left and right and make note where the greatest imbalances lie in those motions. Then treat that problem by working to the "good side." Also, make sure your spiritual, mental, nutritional, and other parts of yourself are in a strong balance.

CHAPTER FOURTEEN

CHIP'S FOUR FAVORITE EXERCISES FOR SHOULDER PAIN PATIENTS

Now comes the fun part! Lab time. Treatment time. Let's put these thoughts into action for your specific shoulder problem. If possible, I would like for you to perform these tests and treatments even as you work through this chapter. Each of these four exercises will be performed following the process below.

1. **TEST** out the motion and compare moving left to moving to the right. You are feeling for imbalances. Those imbalances can be subtle, like one side is a little tighter, weaker, or has just a slightly less full range of motion. Or those imbalances can be more obvious like one side hurts and the other side does not. **Figure out which side is more restricted, AKA the "bad side" and which is better, AKA the "good side."** Even healthy people almost always have one side that is more restricted. You should be able to find a "good" and "bad".

2. **TREATMENT** is then performed by **ONLY** working in the direction of the **GOOD SIDE**. For the sake of this book, this means moving in and out of that "good side" motion for 2 minutes. In the clinic, this prescription can vary.

(Important note: If BOTH SIDES ARE PAINFUL in your test, you skip that exercise altogether and move on to the next one.)

3. After the 2 minutes are completed, go back and **RETEST the "Bad side."** On the retest, figure out if that "bad side" test feels better, unchanged, or worse than the previous time you tested it.

   If better, you might want to continue to work the "good side" until you are fatigued or fixed for now.

   If you are unchanged or worse, before moving on to the next exercise, try that first one with some type of variation. Maybe you hold that exercise longer (like 10-20 seconds), stretch it, change to faster or slower, stand up or sit down, etc. Then after trying the variation, retest the "bad side" again. Sometimes the variation works better than the original version.

If an exercise is helpful, it would be wise to continue doing that exercise over the next days and weeks until hopefully you achieve balance in the testing again.

If those steps do not make perfect sense to you yet, do not sweat it. I will walk you through them one at a time below with each of the four exercises.

Exercise #1: TMR THUMB DOWN SIDE ARM RAISE

This exercise is especially helpful to align the spine and fix strain in the muscles in the upper back, shoulder blade, and shoulder joint regions.

Test out this motion and compare the left side to the right side.

Begin by taking your left arm out to the side and point your thumb to the floor as in picture below.

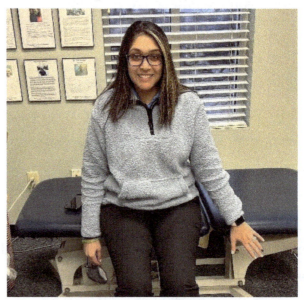

Starting position on the left side

Next, try to raise that left arm up to your side as high as you can, keeping the thumb pointed downward. Preferably, "healthy" would be if the arm could comfortably get all the way behind the head.

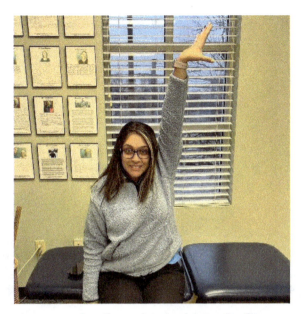

An example of a patient trying to do the test

If this is not the case and is not healthy, make note where the arm stopped and what stopped the motion, like tightness, pain, weakness, or any other factors.

Then perform the same test on the right arm. Make a note as to which arm is the harder one to raise up. Which is the "bad side" and which is the "good side."

We call it an out of balance test when one arm is more restricted.

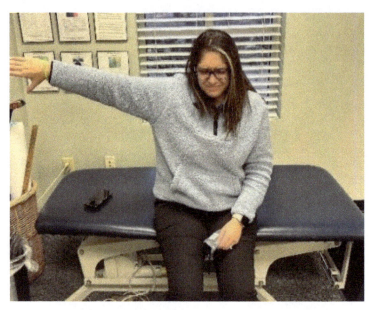

Out of balance test, worse on the right arm

Special note of caution: IF BOTH ARMS ARE NOTICEABLY PAINFUL, do not perform this exercise at all. You can move on to the second one. Otherwise, continue with the exercise.

Once you have measured and felt the "bad arm" on this test, you are going to exercise only the exact same arm motion but using the GOOD SIDE ARM ONLY! For example, if the right arm was the more painful side as in our picture, you are only going to exercise the left arm.

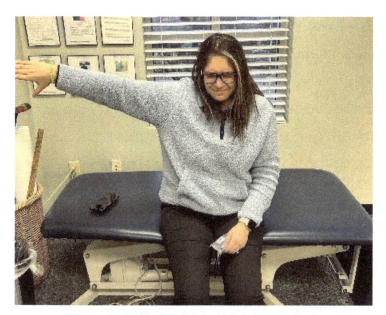

Problem more on right

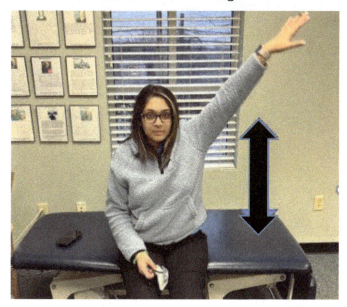

Exercise more on the left

Remember, the purpose of working the "good side" is to try and pull the out of alignment/out of balanced muscles and bones back to where they belong.

Exercise prescription: Lift the "good arm only" up and down to the same thumb down side arm raise exercise for **2 minutes**. Make sure you are stretching as high as you comfortably can with this exercise to not only just work the arm and shoulder, but also to stretch out your ribs, spine, hip, and other areas as best you can as in the picture below. You can do this standing or sitting.

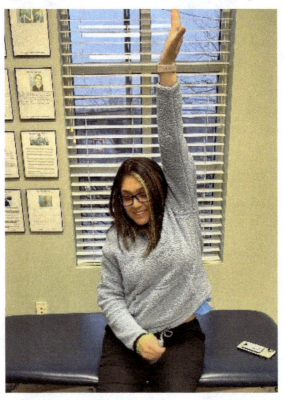

Once you have completed the 2-minute exercise on your "good arm," the next step is to retest the "bad arm" to see if the exercise helped you. Improvements could take the form of less pain, higher range of motion, less clicking, less weakness, or other ways.

So go ahead now and retest the "bad arm." Did this exercise help?

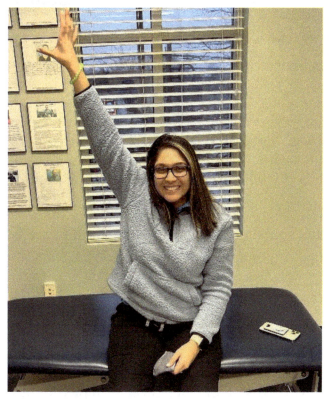

Here she is showing improvement

If you noticed improvement, repeat this exercise throughout today, this week and beyond as long as you see it helping. If you did not notice even a slight positive change, you may want to seek out clinical help as this exercise typically helps close to 95% of the patients I try this with on the first time.

For a video version of this exercise on YouTube, use this link:

https://www.youtube.com/watch?v=GtsMjtnmdZA

Or you can also search YouTube under: "Favorite shoulder pain exercise Chip Moseley".

Exercise #2: TMR BODY TWIST

The body twist exercise is especially helpful to align and balance out the muscles in the mid to lower spine. If you can improve this spinal area, you can then check to see if that gain also benefits your shoulder problem.

Test out the body twist motion and compare the left side to the right side.

Begin by sitting down, touching your knees together, and place your arms crossed on your chest as in picture below.

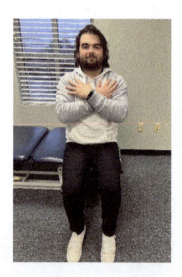

Next, try to twist and rotate your body to the left, while keeping your knees still. A healthy test would be rotating about as far as the picture below with it feeling relatively smooth and easy.

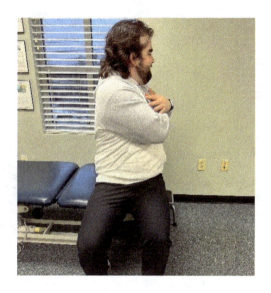

Healthy test for left body twist

Compare the left body twist to the right body twist. Decide which direction is more restricted than the other.

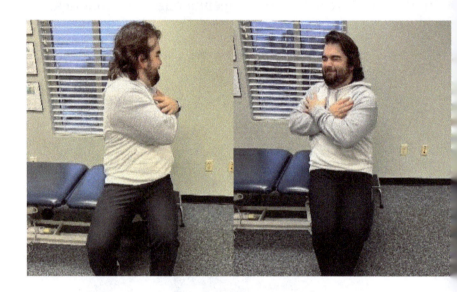

Out of balance test for body twist (worse in right rotation)

Note that even healthy people have one side that is more restricted than the other. For a shoulder pain patient, the differences probably will not be that one side of your body twist "hurts" more than the other. The difference will usually be found that one side is tighter feeling than the other or just cannot move as far as the other side in the range of motion. Now test it out and figure out which side is the harder one to move.

Special note of caution: IF BOTH BODY TWISTS ARE NOTICEABLY PAINFUL, do not perform this next exercise at all. You can move on to exercise number three in the chapter.

Once you have measured and felt the "BAD SIDE" on this twist test, the exercise that you are going to perform is the exact same twist, but using the GOOD SIDE motion only.

Exercise prescription: Twist your body to the "good side only" for **2 minutes**. Make sure you are pushing as far as you comfortably can with this exercise as in picture below.

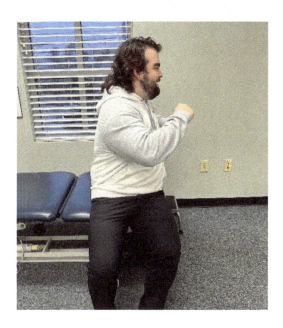

About 1 out of every 20 people will notice during this exercise that their ribs might want to spasm. If this is you, try slumping your back forward a little bit and continue doing the exercise like in the picture below. This should help to lessen that rib strain.

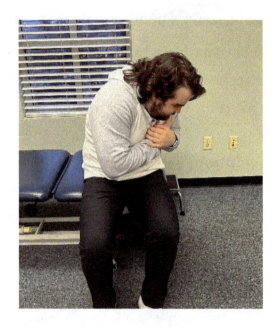

Once you have completed those 2 minutes on your "good side" twist, the next step is to retest the "bad twist" to see if the exercise helped you. Improvements could take the form of less pain, less tightness, greater range of motion, or other ways.

Did this exercise help your spine to twist farther on the "bad side?" If yes, remember that this is an exercise that is helpful for your spine.

After this step is completed, we also add one extra test. This is because we do not only want to know if the twist exercise helped your spine, we also want to know if the twist helped you with your shoulder problem as well. So now go back to the "bad arm" side arm raise thumb down test from the previous exercise

#1 as in picture below. Recheck it again. Did the twist help your arm to feel and move better as well? If yes, then you know that this exercise is also important to continue for your shoulder problem.

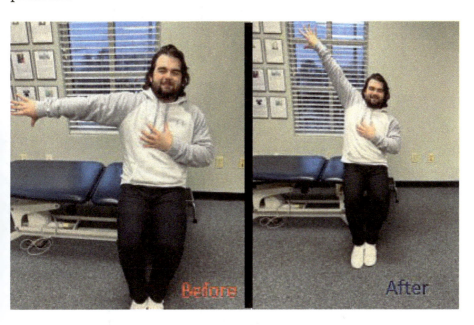

If you noticed improvement in the spine and/or shoulder, repeat this exercise throughout today, this week, and beyond as long as it is helping you.

Exercise #3: TMR LEG RAISE

The leg raise exercise is especially helpful to align and balance out the muscles in the lower spine, hip and pelvic regions. If you are able to improve that area, you can also check to see the exercise has benefits for your shoulder problem.

Test out the leg raise motion and compare the left side to the right side. Begin by sitting down, stretch your left leg out straight in front of you on the ground with a straight knee. Sit up as tall and straight as you can as in the picture below.

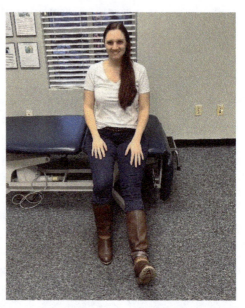

Next, from this starting position, keeping your spine tall and not leaning backwards, lift your left leg up as high as you can. A healthy test would be comfortable with the height of your toes reaching approximately the height of your shoulder.

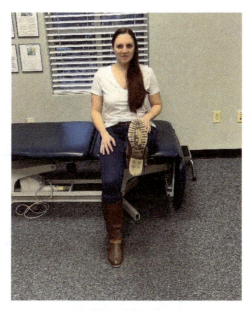

Example of patient trying left leg raise test

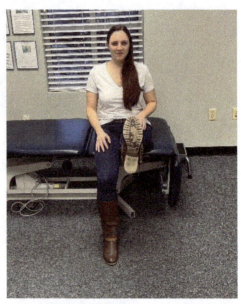

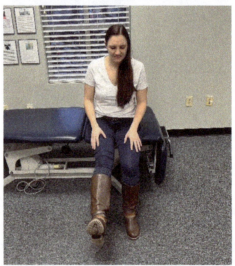

Out of balance test for leg raise, worse on the right side

As with the previous exercises, it is important to note that even healthy people have one side that is more restricted than the other with the leg raise. For a shoulder pain patient, the differences probably will not be that one side hurts more than the other. The difference will usually be found that one side is tighter or weaker/heavier feeling than the other. Possibly one leg just feels more strain in the thigh, cannot raise as high, or is harder to hold up for several seconds. Go ahead and figure out right now which side is the harder one to lift.

Special note of caution again: IF BOTH LEG RAISES ARE NOTICEABLY PAINFUL, do not perform this next exercise at all. If both sides HURT, you can move on to Exercise #4. Otherwise continue.

Once you have measured and felt the "BAD SIDE" on this leg raise test, as mentioned in previous parts of this book, the exercise that you are going to perform is the exact same motion, but using the GOOD SIDE LEG RAISE only!

Exercise prescription: Raise your leg to the "good side only" for **2 minutes**. Make sure you are pushing as far as you comfortably can with this exercise as in picture below. You can either do repetitions up and down quickly, slowly, or hold it in the air for a few seconds at a time. You can even let your hands help you a little if needed. Feel free to rest here and there for a few seconds if you need the rest. But work the "good side" leg raise for the full 2 minutes.

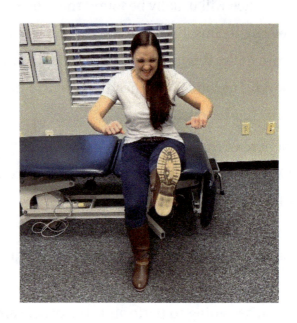

Once you have completed those 2 minutes on your "good side" leg raise, the next step is to retest the "bad side" leg raise to see if the exercise helped your lower back, pelvic, and hip region. Improvements could take the form of less pain, less tightness, greater range of motion, a stronger feel, or other ways.

Did this exercise help your leg raise on the "bad side"? If yes, remember that this is an exercise that is helpful for your lower spine, hip, and pelvic region.

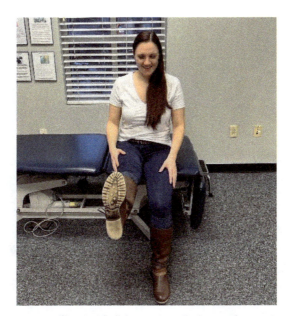

Retest "bad side" leg raise. Is it any better?

After you rechecked the leg raise, you can now go back to retest the shoulder again by retesting the bad arm with the side arm raise with the thumb down as in picture below. Do this now. Did the leg raise help your "bad" arm to feel and move better too? If yes, then you know that this exercise is also important to continue for your shoulder problem.

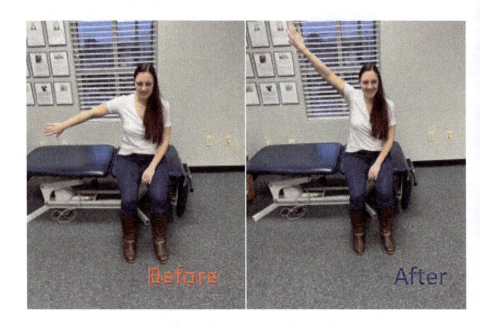

If you noticed improvement in the leg raise test and/or shoulder, repeat this exercise throughout today, this week and beyond as long as you see it helping you.

Exercise #4: TMR SIDE ARM PRESS ON THE WALL

The side arm press exercise is especially helpful to align and balance out the muscles in the upper to middle spine and shoulder blade regions.

Test out the left side arm press on the wall. Begin by standing up and reach your left arm out to the side on the wall at about shoulder height. Hand and wrist should be in a neutral and comfortable position.

Next, from this starting position, lean your body weight towards the wall as your elbow bends as in picture on the next page. I think of this as if I am doing a sideways push up on the wall. A healthy test would be a strong lean to the wall from a larger distance off the wall. Feel free to move closer to the wall if the first distance is too difficult or further from the wall if this test is too easy. To do an even higher level, try doing a push up on the floor with more weight on one arm.

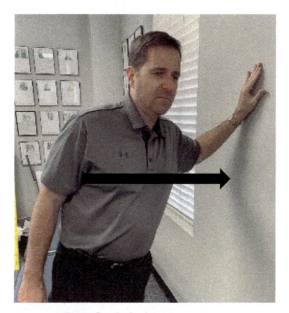

Test for left side arm press

Compare the left side arm press on the wall to the right side arm press. Which arm is harder to lean on?

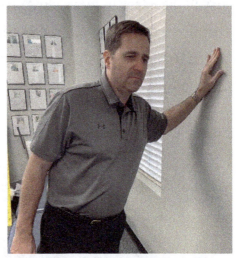

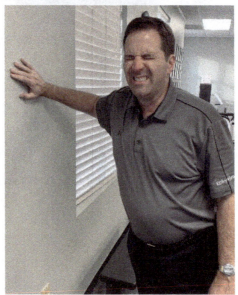

Out of balance test for side arm press on the wall, worse on the right

For a shoulder pain patient, the injured arm, or "bad side" might be limited by pain, tightness, weakness, or other factors. Go ahead now and figure out which side is the harder one to move.

Special note of caution again: IF BOTH SIDE ARM PRESSES ARE NOTICEABLY PAINFUL, do not perform this next exercise at all. Just focus on the previous exercises in choices 1-3 that were helpful for you.

Once you have measured and felt the "BAD SIDE" on this arm press test, go exercise the exact same motion, but using the GOOD SIDE ARM PRESS only!

Exercise prescription: Perform the side arm press on the wall on the "good side only" for **2 minutes**. Make sure you are leaning as far as you comfortably can with this exercise.

Once you have completed those 2 minutes on your "good side" arm press, go back and retest the "bad side" arm press. Was the test any better? Improvements could take the form of less pain, less tightness, greater range of motion, a stronger feel, or other forms.

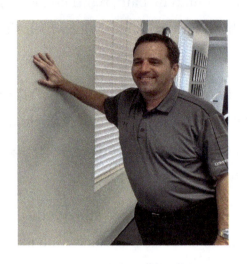

Did this exercise help your shoulder problem? If yes, repeat this exercise throughout today, this week, and beyond as long as you see it helping you.

Key Thought #14: Try out Chip's four favorite shoulder exercises using our TMR Principles. Whichever ones help the most, continue performing them for the next days and weeks as long as you see progress.

CHAPTER FIFTEEN

HOW LONG DOES IT TAKE TO GET MY SHOULDER BETTER?

WILL THE EXERCISE BENEFITS LAST?

Almost every shoulder patient who comes into our clinic leaves after the first visit feeling and moving at least a little bit better than when they came in. Obviously, lesser injuries show greater early improvements than deeper injuries. While we expect early gains even on day one, the next question is, "How long will those gains last?" We tend to attract a lot of patients that have been to several other professionals that did not "fix them," but who came to us because they heard we have some newer ideas. Those patients who struggled to show improvement elsewhere are typically very excited to see "something different" that seemed to be beneficial on day one. But they are also typically and understandably suspicious that such gains will not last as they have seen in the past from other treatments.

So how can you make the gains last? Or another question might be why does one patient seem to do treatment and keep those gains to apply to the next session, while another patient can be feeling like they are back to square one just a short time after walking out of our door where they just made noticeable gains?

Over all of my years of being a clinician, I have only figured out four potential reasons why the gains made on the shoulder of one person can be brief while others have gains that seem to last longer.

Reason #1 why pain can return later:

PROPRIOCEPTORS KEEPING THE STATUS QUO

A benefit to our active exercise treatments is that improvements made in the shoulder and other parts of the body were made by the patient doing something on themselves and not by a passive treatment done by the therapist on them. As mentioned in Chapter Ten, I can still be a big fan of passive treatments such as massage, chiropractic, acupuncture, and other such options, but what is the flaw in those treatments? The flaw is that the clinician, no matter how skilled or effective, does not go home with the patient! That becomes a problem since the body tends to naturally resist changes, especially at first. If the problem returns, that clinician is not at home with that patient to repeat the treatment.

The body is full of nerve endings called *proprioceptors*. To us anatomy geeks, these proprioceptors have names such as muscle spindles, Golgi tendon organs, Golgi ligament organs, Ruffini endings, mechano-joint receptors, and others.

What is the job of these nerve endings? Their job is basically to **keep the "status quo."** This status quo might be linked to certain joint alignment, muscle tension/ lengths, movement patterns, postures, or other factors.

When you are healthy, these proprioceptors work in your favor. Let us say, for example, that you have been pretty pain free without trauma for most of your life. But then you do a "weekend warrior" task in your yard and now your shoulder has pain. If this is the case, you will most likely find that a few days later, your shoulder is back to pain free again. This is due to the body reverting to its baseline, which previously was in a pretty healthy condition.

However, in a contrasting example, let us say that many years ago, you had an injury moment in your body. As previously mentioned, this injury leads to tissues tightening around that area, bones changing their alignments, and other changes that factor in to how your shoulder and body presents today. So, when you perform these treatments like the exercises from the previous chapter, the body is in better balance, the muscles are in more proper lengths, and you have less pain and better function at that moment.

However, a few hours later, what is starting to happen? The body is reverting back to its "status quo." In this case, that means reverting back to its injured position with joint alignment, muscular tension, and so forth from the "old injuries." Gains made in the clinic at first are typically resisted as the body tries to go back to this previous state. Furthermore, this moment of improvement followed by a moment of reversion back to baseline often causes muscular soreness, even in areas where that person might not be typically sore. This soreness can be discouraging if you are not expecting it. The good news is that the soreness tends to get less and less over time with treatment. Kind of like this dog below, we have to train it to "stay!"

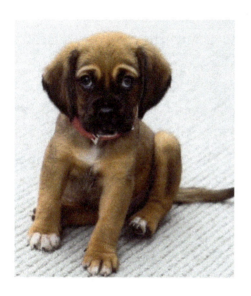

While we expect this resistance at first from this status quo, what is the good news for the person who made themselves better using our exercises? The good news is that while the clinician does not go home with those patients, their arms, bodies and legs do go with them wherever they go!

So, the lesson is that if you continue making the body better through the exercises at home, you can win the war! Make it last. **Fix the system to fix the symptoms.**

Have you ever heard how long it takes to "change a habit?" Depending on the research you read, the answer lies somewhere in the twenty-one days to two-month range in most studies. How does this "change" occur? It happens because of these aforementioned proprioceptors! They can learn. They can change. They can learn to "stay" like a good dog. Whatever tissue position, length, or other factor you can keep that bone, muscle, or other soft tissue looking like for about a month or two, you can make it stick and change to that new place! This is basically establishing the "new normal" by reprogramming these proprioceptors.

The secret to fixing the proprioceptors is CONSISTENT AND FREQUENT TREATMENT. This might mean spreading the exercises out and performing them several times a day instead of just once or twice a day. Keep working those treatment exercises until they stick, and the tests look "in balance."

Reason #2 why pain can return later:

THE DEPTH OF THE INJURY

Another reason why pain can return later for some is that the injury itself may have been deeper and more significant than the injury of others. Compare a shoulder pain that happened due to a poor postural use of a computer mouse to a patient that got hit by a giant truck going 80 mph! The first patient can have pain. But the second patient has muscle and joint injuries that might be significantly deeper.

As you might imagine, it would take higher force and probably longer term treatments to fix the deeper injury than it is to fix the lesser deep problem. So you have to dig deeper!

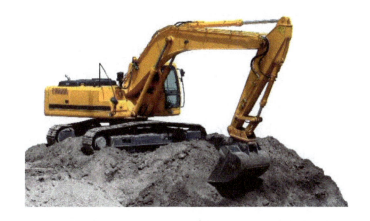

The secret to fixing the deeper injuries is DEEPER FORMS OF TREATMENT. This might mean doing more repetitions, more time, more weight, or more force on the exercises to get the result than what the lighter injured patient might need.

Reason #3 why pain can return later:

POSTURES AND DAILY LIFE CHOICES THAT FEED THE INJURY

I still remember one patient like it was yesterday. For the sake of the book, I will call him Dave. While it seems more recent to me, technically it was back in 2008 when Dave was being treated in our clinic. He had chronic low back pain that had plagued him for years. He had seen many clinicians and tried many treatments that never gave him even a moment of relief. The good news is that after his first two sessions on week one,

Dave felt about 20% better. This was dramatic for a guy who had never had one moment of relief as aforementioned.

Then came that next early Monday morning... Oh boy... Dave came in the door with an attitude. He tracked me down and in front of about five other patients, succeeded to yell at me for about 15 minutes about how horrible his back pain was and that our treatments made him worse, and we would never be able to fix his problem. While no one enjoys being yelled at, I did let him continue until the volume dropped a little and I then proceeded to ask him a couple of poignant questions.

The conversation went something like this...

CHIP: "Dave, I remember when you did that body twist exercise last week, your pain would almost always go down in a way that was very significant. Did you do that body twist exercise as discussed over the weekend?"

DAVE: "Yes."

CHIP: "How often did you do that exercise? I know we discussed doing it for about twenty to thirty minutes a day if not more."

DAVE: "I only did one set of the exercise for 3 minutes once a day. I did not do any more than that."

CHIP: "Alright, Dave, you did something. Not as often as we discussed, but you did do something. How did your pain feel when you did that exercise?"

DAVE: "I could tell it felt better, but the relief definitely did not last. And as I said, I feel even worse after the weekend!"

CHIP: "Gotcha, Dave. I have one more question. What did you do the rest of the weekend during those 23 hours and 57 minutes each day that you were not doing your exercises?"

DAVE: "Actually, Chip. You would have been very impressed with me. For 10 hours on Saturday and 10 hours on Sunday I WAS CHOPPING WOOD!"

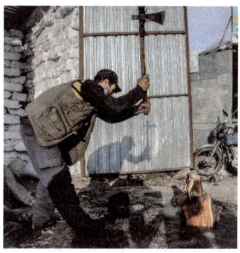

At this point, not only did I almost fall out of my chair, but you could also see almost every other patient in the room roll their eyes back and let out a groan. Because obviously, while this story apparently was not blatantly obvious to Dave, he was chopping wood for many hours that was straining his back injury, while only doing three minutes a day of his exercise that was healing to him.

We think of it as a giant old-timey scale. On one side of the scale, you have postures, actions, and activities that are healing for the body. On the other side, you have those same factors that are feeding the injury.

Have you ever wondered why you can have a "good day" with your pain on Tuesday followed by a "bad day" with your pain on Wednesday? The simple answer is that on the "bad day," the scale weighed heavier on the 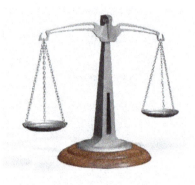 actions that promoted the injury. On the "good day," the scale weighed heavier on the side that promoted healing.

The secret to fixing these issues is to identify and **FIX THE SOURCE OF POSTURAL OR ACTIVITY STRAIN**. This means to change those postures and motions of strain to positions that are more comfortable and less tense and forceful on the injury.

Most cases are not as obvious as "Dave." This source of strain may lie in the chair we sit in at our computer. Is the chair the right height? Does it possess the right amount of cushion? Is it better to have a tall or slouchy posture in that chair? There are times that slouchy is better and times where tall is better, depending on the injury. How about sleeping postures?

Most patients tend to choose postures that they assume are correct, like sitting up tall, for example. However, some injuries are worse when someone sits up really straight! That person would heal better when slouched. So, if that person tries to sit up tall in that example, doing what was assumed to be correct is actually feeding the injury. It is better for healing to be in the most comfortable and least amount of tension and energy consuming postures.

Reason #4 why pain can return later:

THE MISSING PIECE

We have discussed how the body is a bunch of connected tissues together of bones, muscles, fascia, and other items that influence each other. Because of this, I can have a bone that is off in my foot that then changes my knee, followed by my hip and back, and that reaction keeps going until before I know it, I have a really bad migraine headache. Or it could be the other way around. I could have a problem in my neck that changes my shoulder, then spine, and before I know it, I can have a foot pain.

Since one problem can lead to another, it is important to not only fix the areas of symptoms, but also to fix the source of the symptoms. This can be very tricky especially for those who are not trained to **fix the system to fix the symptoms**. If I went back to physical therapy school again tomorrow or attended medical school, nursing school, and many other sources of education, most clinicians are typically trained to address the area of the injury exclusively. In other words, if you have a shoulder problem, we only test and treat the shoulder area itself. Some schools may briefly recommend that you consider looking close to the area of injury, but rarely is it taught in education that you MUST **look at the system to fix the symptoms** as I am suggesting.

As a result, even if a clinician is effective at improving a problem in one area like the shoulder, it will be frustrating to the patient when that problem consistently returns because you have not fixed the mechanical source elsewhere. You have not fixed the system.

Other missing pieces that can cause shoulder pains may include issues that are not just muscle and bone related. If someone had a tumor in their upper lung, for example, then they might also have pain in the shoulder area as well. Keep in mind, this is very rare. I do not want you to feel that you need to go have your lungs examined with an MRI just because you have shoulder pain. But if this is the source, the pain will not go away until you fix the problem.

Emotional, mental, and spiritual issues can also create tensions that can create a shoulder pain and keep it from getting healed. I will never forget treating this lady back in 2006. For the sake of the book, I will call her Stacy. Stacy had a frozen shoulder/adhesive capsulitis and she could barely raise her arm off her hip for years. Radiology was clean. Several clinicians and doctors before me had never been able to help her even a little.

Over the first 3-4 weeks of clinical treatment, I was right in line with the results of her previous clinicians. I had not helped her at all even with trying both newer and older treatment options to various intensities. She had me stumped. One day I decided that if I was not able to improve her on her next scheduled session, I would discharge her from our clinic since I was not helping her.

She arrived to this session unaware of my plans to possibly finish her therapy. When I was taking her back to the treatment area, she asked if we could go to a private room because she had something to tell me. When I took her back to the room, she started crying very forcefully for several minutes, at first unable to speak. Once she could start talking in a manner I could understand, she explained that her husband had gotten ill a few years back and he never would speak to her anymore during the day. Furthermore, since she had to take care of him, it was difficult to get out of the house and she had lost contact with friends and family over the years. As a result, she was basically very lonely and sad. After we continued talking for about twenty minutes, she told me she was thankful she had me to talk to and unload her problems. She thought I was a nice enough guy and she needed to "get it out" to someone. I told her I was glad to be there for her and I would pray for her. After this was done, I asked her to start our official session itself by showing me how high she could raise up her arm.

To my shock, she raised her arm fully over her head and pain free! I almost fell out of my chair. Apparently, her frozen shoulder was not physical. It was the emotional stress and sadness that occurred from her last few years of issues with husband and *her life's* circumstances. The treatment for Stacy's shoulder was for her to keep finding people she could talk to about her problems and try to get some semblance of a social life back to normal. **Fix the system to fix the symptoms**.

What is the secret to fixing the missing piece?

Identify and fix the source of trhe problem, even if that means looking into places you would not normally expect.

Key Thought #15: To make sure your shoulder problem stays fixed for good, you need to address the proprioceptors that try to keep the status quo, the depth of the injury, the postures and actions that feed the injury, and the missing pieces through fixing the system.

CHAPTER SIXTEEN

WHAT TREATMENT LOOKS LIKE IN OUR CLINIC

At Total Motion Physical Therapy in Raleigh, we strive to give world class quality care with the focus on the principles that have been discussed in this book. On the first session, I tell each new patient that we basically have three goals for any patient who walks into our doors.

1. **Fix the symptoms.** (Pain, tightness, weakness, lack of functional range of motion, etc.)
2. **Fix the CAUSE of the symptoms.** This means fixing the mechanics that feed the problem as we have discussed in the book. Identify the tight injured areas outside of the shoulder that also need addressing and fix them as well.
3. **Empower our patient with the skills** on how to use a tool we created here called **TMR**, Total Motion Release, so they can learn how to become their own clinician and fix their own pains.

It is really the second and third goals that set us apart from your typical other clinics that treat shoulder pain. There are many treatment options out there that can decrease a pain for a period of time. However, there are very few clinicians that know how to find and fix the mechanical source of the problem by identifying the areas of tightness and weakness in the system. And most of all, being the source site of the creation of Total Motion Release (TMR), our clinic goes far beyond just "I'm making you feel good right now." We are big fans of the "teach a man to fish and he can feed himself for life" versus the "give a man a fish and feed him for a day" philosophy. If you make the pain go down but do not fix the source, it will come back again. If you have only been treated by someone else doing a treatment on you, you have to keep going back and back to that same clinician to do the "trick" to feel better. If you know how to test and fix your own problems, you can address any issue that may arise in the future.

This book is just the tip of the iceberg on how to get started at treating yourself or others using our principles. I gave four exercises that act as a springboard to start you on a journey of fixing.

The fun part is that we all should have 206 bones, around 600 muscles, and a presentation that is unique to each of us. Each person who walks in our door has had a multitude of moments of life unique to them that presents in their bodies in a unique way. Technically, we will never see the same patient twice. We will treat a lot of "shoulder impingement" syndromes, but what the shoulder, neck, spine, hip, and other parts of each person's body look like that are part of that injury will be different with each individual. Those differences are magnified when combined with different personalities, walks of life, job choices, social goals, and other factors. Each patient presents to us a fun journey and individual puzzle to solve that goes from day one to getting them back to normal.

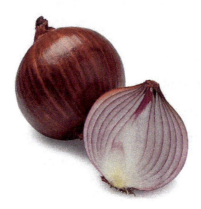

In many cases, I may have a really good idea what the outcome would be for that person, but our joyful challenge is to get them to "go on that journey" with us to get them to where they want to be. Sometimes the therapy is not that complicated, but the person might be very complicated in other ways. In other cases, someone may have many compounding injuries and one week can look very different from the next. The more complicated cases are also fun to start on that journey, although it is harder to predict how next week's presentation might look like. Like the onion, there are many "layers" of injury and we peel them back one layer at a time until there is nothing left to peel!

As a result of our specific clinical goals and background, our therapy is very active with mostly using certain exercises, motions, and postures to teach our patients how to fix themselves. We do not focus nearly as much on machines, modalities, and manual therapy like many others might. If I feel that any of those other options might be helpful in a case, I will often refer out to an appropriate clinician to perform those tasks while we work on the strategy that we are performing. We prefer the active treatments so that each patient can treat themselves to a natural fix. "Teach a man to fish."

Key Thought #16: In our clinic, the three goals of therapy are to fix the symptoms, fix the mechanical cause of the symptoms, and to empower our patients on how to take care of their own pains through using our tool, TMR.

CHAPTER SEVENTEEN

SUMMARIZING IT ALL – A REVIEW OF THE KEY PRINCIPLES

Key Thought #1: Shoulder pain can severely affect how you enjoy life. Seeking out proper treatment quickly is critical to getting your life back.

Key Thought #2: Choosing the wrong treatment or waiting longer to address the problem can make the shoulder injury worse and more difficult to properly treat.

Key Thought #3: If you can do actions that make the pain go up, then you have a musculoskeletal issue and there are actions you can do to make the pain go down.

Key Thought #4: Understanding how the anatomy of the rotator cuff works will start you on the journey of knowing how to fix your shoulder pain.

Key Thought #5: Shoulder pain is caused by tightness in the body that changes the mechanics of how the arm would normally move. This tightness can originate from any place in the body.

Key Thought #6: You must see the tightness in the system to fix the symptoms.

Key Thought #7: Having a larger amount of body parts that can move well, especially in the power zones, leads to less strain on the shoulder and thus greater healing.

Key Thought #8: Most of the time you can start a therapy program without having radiology done on the shoulder. Radiology is most helpful when there is extreme trauma or concern that a surgery is needed instead of conservative treatment.

Key Thought #9: Barring a trauma, tightness in the system is what causes the five different types of shoulder injury. The five different shoulder injuries are: impingement, partial rotator cuff tear, full rotator cuff tear, adhesive capsulitis, and instability.

Key Thought #10: The traditional flow of treatment options in medicine for shoulder pain has flaws. It is best to start with a movement specialist like a PT who can screen and send to others as needed, or choose to start treatment to correct the mechanical problem without unnecessary surgeries or medications.

Key Thought #11: Traditional shoulder stretching and strengthening exercises can add to the injury more than help heal the injury. In order to heal with exercise, you must consider other options.

Key Thought #12: Apply the principles of "TREAT", with constant testing, retesting, and making adjustments as needed in order to get to the desired result in the fastest way possible.

Key Thought #13: A balanced and well aligned system is healthier than one that is out of balance. Test the body by comparing motion to the left and right and make note where the greatest imbalances lie in those motions. Then treat that problem by working to the "good side." Also, make sure your spiritual, mental, nutritional, and other parts of yourself are in a strong balance.

Key Thought #14: Try out Chip's four favorite shoulder exercises using our TMR Principles. Whichever ones help the most, continue performing them for the next days and weeks as long as you see progress.

Key Thought #15: To make sure your shoulder problem stays fixed for good, you need to address the proprioceptors that try to keep the status quo, the depth of the injury, the postures and actions that feed the injury, and the missing pieces through fixing the system.

Key Thought #16: In our clinic, the three goals of therapy are to fix the symptoms, fix the mechanical cause of the symptoms, and to empower our patients on how to take care of their own pains through using our tool, TMR.

CHAPTER EIGHTEEN

SUCCESS STORIES

Below are a few examples of patients who were treated successfully with our TMR therapy at Total Motion Physical Therapy in Raleigh. What did they think about our treatment for their shoulder pains?

1. Keith B.

"I came to Total Motion with serious pain in my right shoulder presumably from weight lifting. When I started, I could hardly lift my right arm above shoulder height in the gym, and struggled with pain throughout the day on a consistent basis. After my initial meeting with Chip, I trusted his assessment and agreed to a 15-session program.

The program, through Chip, Prachi and Jonathan, taught me how to identify problem movements and how to address those problems with targeted exercises. The Total Motion team oversaw my progress and carefully put together a plan to follow while I was there in person and at home.

After 5 short weeks, I am back in the gym, exercising as normal and know how to identify and treat soreness or pain on my own! I trust the Total Motion Team and the program and would be happy to recommend them to anyone with pain that interferes with desired activities or day-to-day life!"

2. Marcia M.

"For about 15 years, I've had on and off pain in my right shoulder, neck and arm and have been to numerous Chiropractors and Physical Therapists; they always got the pain to go away, but it always returned. Two years ago, I injured my left hip and my right side got worse. I spent 6 months with a chiropractor, another 3 months with a PT, and then came across an Instagram post for a shoulder workshop at Total Motion PT. At the workshop, I not only felt release from just a couple of exercises, but learned that I could help myself become pain free. Their concept is completely different than any PT I've been to– working the side that doesn't hurt to heal the side that does! I'm almost pain free and am set with stretches and exercises to keep me that way. Many thanks to Chip and his entire staff. I highly recommend!"

3. Ronald M.

"They were the only ones that worked for me! I had severe shoulder and back pain caused by trying to walk my German Shepherd Dog. My doctor prescribed physical therapy which I took twice a week for eight weeks. I followed that up with 8 weeks of workout at the gym with a private trainer. It was all very fine but did not solve the pain. I still could not raise my left arm above horizontal. A friend then recommended for me to try Total Motion.

I went and am very glad I did. MY PAIN IS GONE! In addition to that great result, they teach you how to stay pain free. While being treated you learn how the body works. It was amazing how their approach reaches every part of the body. After finishing my PT, I returned a few weeks later to measure my progress against what it was when I left. I was even further improving on my own and remained painless. I would recommend them to anyone with pain."

4. Pat P.

"I was considering rotator cuff surgery on my right shoulder. My doc kept saying, 'There are a lot of moving parts in there. You might want to get looked at.' I met with 4 friends who have had the surgery and in all cases, it was more-or-less successful. However, it set each of them back a minimum of 6 months of recovery and another 6 months of therapy. Saw Total Motion on Facebook and clicked on the ad. Then registered for the on-line Zoom assessment. One of the Zoom meeting exercises was to help raise my arm which I could not raise above my shoulder. A few exercises later and I could raise it well above my shoulder...I was sold! Figured it was worth the trial - after a couple of months, I can raise my right arm almost 180 degrees! Crazy!!! The techniques Chip and his team promote are completely off the reservation...but they work!! I wholeheartedly endorse Total Motion PT to ANYONE considering surgery. This saved me from going under the knife! Thanks Chip and Team!!!"

5. Thomas G.

"I went to Total Motion PT for what I thought was a torn rotator cuff. I could only move my left arm about 3 inches from my side. Chip tested my arm and told me it was a severe shoulder impingement. Chip showed me a few exercises to do to see if I had even other issues. Since I had no other problems, he scheduled me for 8 sessions. After 8 sessions, I saw about 80% improvement. HAPPY CAMPER!! I did 6 weeks of therapy and improved 100%–had all of my range of motions and 95% of my strength back. Traditional therapy probably would have taken at least 5-6 months to heal compared to 6 weeks at Total Motion. Chip's theory of treatment and teaching you how to heal yourself is unique, beneficial, self-absorbing and very rewarding. If someone have any issues with body movements, I highly recommend Total Motion PT with Chip Moseley and his wonderful staff."

ABOUT THE AUTHOR

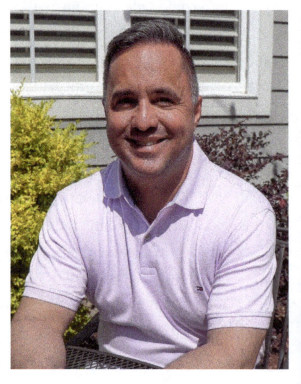

Chip Moseley, MPT is one of the two owners of Total Motion Physical Therapy in Raleigh, NC, along with his business partner, Deanna Merritt. After growing up in Raleigh, Chip got both his Bachelor's Degree in Chemistry and his Master's degree in Physical Therapy from the University of North Carolina at Chapel Hill. Since that time, he has had hundreds of hours in continuing education. Back in the late 1990s in Knoxville, TN, Chip earned his Board Certified Specialist in Orthopedics and Certified Strength and Conditioning Specialist honors.

After returning to Raleigh in 2002, Chip joined up with the owner of Total Motion PT at that time, Tom Dalonzo-Baker. As mentioned in the book above, together with Tom, Total Motion Release, TMR, was created where other clinicians and patients can learn how to fix their own pains. Several years ago, Tom sold the clinic to Chip and his co-owner, Deanna Merritt. Chip has continued with treating patients since that time using the TMR principles and training the next generation to take his place.

Chip presently lives in Rolesville, NC, along with his beautiful wife, Nancy. Chip has four boys, Chase, Jaxon, Brad, and James, and one girl, Molly. Chase and Molly are now married and Chase and his bride, Ashlee, have now given Chip and Nancy their first granddaughter, Charlotte. Jaxon has followed in his Dad's footsteps to UNC-Chapel Hill and the twin boys are in high school.

Chip is also a Sunday School teacher at Faith Baptist Church in Youngsville, NC. He has coached countless basketball and soccer teams over the years, but now enjoys being more of a fan.

You can reach Chip at **chip@tmptnc.com**, or you can reach the clinic at 919.872.2828, 4030 Wake Forest Road, Suite 211, Raleigh, NC, 27609.

CPSIA information can be obtained
at www.ICGtesting.com
Printed in the USA
JSHW010358130723
44439JS00004B/17